ABC of
Dementia

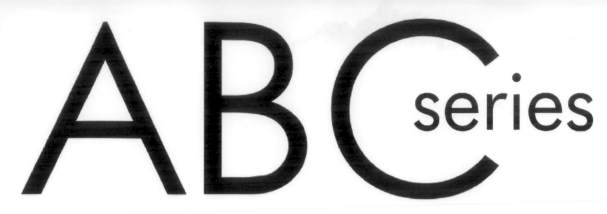

ABC series

An outstanding collection of resources for everyone in primary care

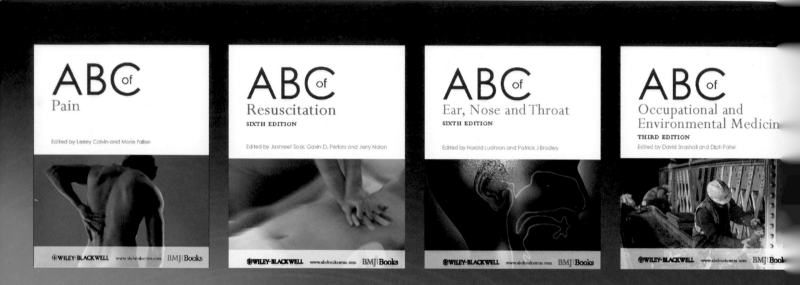

ABC of Pain
Edited by Lesley Colvin and Marie Fallon

ABC of Resuscitation
SIXTH EDITION
Edited by Jasmeet Soar, Gavin D. Perkins and Jerry Nolan

ABC of Ear, Nose and Throat
SIXTH EDITION
Edited by Harold Ludman and Patrick J Bradley

ABC of Occupational and Environmental Medicine
THIRD EDITION
Edited by David Snashall and Dipti Patel

The *ABC* series contains a wealth of indispensable resources for GPs, GP registrars, junior doctors, doctors in training and all those in primary care

▶ **Highly illustrated, informative and a practical source of knowledge**

▶ **An easy-to-use resource, covering the symptoms, investigations, treatment and management of conditions presenting in day-to-day practice and patient support**

▶ **Full colour photographs and illustrations aid diagnosis and patient understanding of a condition**

For more information on all books in the *ABC* series, including links to further information, references and links to the latest official guidelines, please visit:

www.abcbookseries.com

✦WILEY-BLACKWELL

BMJ|Books

ABC of Dementia

EDITED BY

Bernard Coope, MBChB, MMedSci, MRCPsych

Associate Medical Director, Consultant Older Adult Psychiatrist
Worcestershire Health and Care NHS Trust

Felicity A. Richards, MBChB, MRCPsych, DGM

Consultant Older Adult Psychiatrist
Worcestershire Health and Care NHS Trust

WILEY Blackwell   BMJ Books

This edition first published 2014 © 2014 by John Wiley & Sons Ltd.

BMJ Books is an imprint of BMJ Publishing Group Limited, used under licence by John Wiley & Sons.

Registered office: John Wiley & Sons, Ltd, The Atrium, Southern Gate, Chichester, West Sussex, PO19 8SQ, UK

Editorial offices: 9600 Garsington Road, Oxford, OX4 2DQ, UK

The Atrium, Southern Gate, Chichester, West Sussex, PO19 8SQ, UK

111 River Street, Hoboken, NJ 07030-5774, USA

For details of our global editorial offices, for customer services and for information about how to apply for permission to reuse the copyright material in this book please see our website at www.wiley.com/wiley-blackwell

The right of the author to be identified as the author of this work has been asserted in accordance with the UK Copyright, Designs and Patents Act 1988.

Library of Congress Cataloging-in-Publication Data

ABC of dementia / edited by Bernie Coope and Felicity A. Richards.
    p. ; cm.
  Includes bibliographical references and index.
  ISBN 978-1-118-47402-0 (pbk.)
  I. Coope, Bernie, 1964– editor. II. Richards, Felicity A. (Felicity Ann), 1979– editor.   [DNLM: 1. Dementia – diagnosis – Great Britain.
2. Dementia – therapy – Great Britain. WM 220]
  RC521
  616.8′3 – dc23

2013046742

A catalogue record for this book is available from the British Library.

Wiley also publishes its books in a variety of electronic formats. Some content that appears in print may not be available in electronic books.

Cover image: iStockphoto.com/stevecoleimages
Cover design by Meaden Creative

Set in 9.25/12 MinionPro by Laserwords Private Ltd, Chennai, India
Printed and bound in Malaysia by Vivar Printing Sdn Bhd

2   2015

Contents

List of Contributors

Peter Bentham
Birmingham Memory Assessment and Rare Dementia Services, Birmingham, UK

Dawn Brooker
Association for Dementia Studies, University of Worcester, Worcester, UK

Bernard Coope
Worcestershire Health and Care NHS Trust, Worcestershire, UK

Tanya Jacobs
Worcestershire Health and Care NHS Trust, Worcestershire, UK

Jelena Jankovic
Dudley and Walsall Mental Health Partnership Trust, Dudley, UK

Jenny La Fontaine
Association for Dementia Studies, University of Worcester, Henwick Grove, Worcester, UK

Daryl L. Leung
Elderly Care and Dementia Service Royal Wolverhampton NHS Trust, Wolverhampton, UK

Dhanjeev Marrie
Worcestershire Health and Care NHS Trust, Worcestershire, UK

Felicity A. Richards
Worcestershire Health and Care NHS Trust, Worcestershire, UK

Simon Rumley
Aylmer Lodge Cookley Partnership, Kidderminster, Worcestershire, UK

Solmaz Sadaghiani
Worcestershire Health and Care NHS Trust, Worcestershire, UK

Georgios Theodoulou
Worcestershire Health and Care NHS Trust, Worcestershire, UK

Kay de Vries
Graduate School of Nursing, Midwifery & Health (GSNMH), Victoria University of Wellington, NZ; Association for Dementia Studies, University of Worcester, UK, University of Washington, Seattle, USA

Elizabeth Ward
Royal Wolverhampton NHS Trust, Wolverhampton, UK

Sally Williams
Worcestershire Health and Care NHS Trust, Worcestershire, UK

Introduction–A Call to Action

Bernard Coope and Felicity A. Richards

Worcestershire Health and Care NHS Trust, Worcestershire, UK

Historically, dementia has not featured highly in the training of either medical students or junior doctors. Dementia is now gaining increasing recognition as a health care issue in it's own right. The field of dementia care is transforming rapidly (Figure 1), and whatever the area of health care you are involved in, you will at some point be touched by dementia. With this comes the need for all clinicians to learn about dementia. It is hoped that this book will play its part in helping clinicians understand the evolving nature of the evidence base, changes in societal expectations and the effects dementia has on the person, their family and the health service.

Why is the need to learn about dementia changing?

The evidence base

The past two decades have seen a rapid growth in the scientific understanding of dementia and the brain diseases that cause it, including developments in neuropathology, aetiology, imaging and the role of genetics. In turn, this knowledge led to the introduction of pharmacological treatments and, consequently, an evidence base for their limited effectiveness. As yet, no available treatments modify the brain diseases causing dementia and there is no evidence to support screening programmes.

Continued research has also led to the discovery that many of the treatments that have been used for decades with the clinical aim of helping people with dementia do more harm than good. Sedating treatments such as antipsychotics are of little clinical effectiveness and are known to increase mortality in those patients prescribed them. Fortunately, we are moving away from pharmacological treatments towards a range of non-medical interventions to help those most distressed or most challenging to care for. Central to this has been the flourishing of research and theory in the field of person-centred care.

A final illustration of the changing evidence base is the demonstration of the effectiveness of service interventions. Supporting carers by providing information and emotional support can prolong a carer's ability to provide care at home, reducing the need for a move to longer term placement. A well-made and well-communicated early diagnosis, backed up by post-diagnostic support, can improve the quality of care for the person with dementia and their families, as well as reducing the risk of crises in the future.

Changes in society

Dementia is a condition that gets commoner with age. More than half of those with dementia in the UK are over 80. It is this age group that is growing in countries across the world and with this growth, the number of people with dementia is climbing.

As the number of people with dementia has been rising, the structure of families has been changing. Close members of the family have traditionally stepped in to provide care for people with dementia, with the majority of carers being either spouses or daughters. There is an increasing trend for people to enter old age separated and for children to be living at a greater distance from their parents and to be in full time work. The capacity of family members to take on a caring role will have an impact on what is expected from professionals in health and social care.

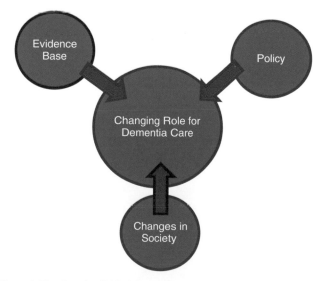

Figure 1 The changing field of dementia care.

Box 1 Dementia Action Alliance: Call to Action

1. I have personal choice and control or influence over decisions about me

- I have control over my life and support to do the things that matter to me.
- I have received an early diagnosis, which was sensitively communicated.
- I have access to adequate resources (private and public) that enable me to choose where and how I live.
- I can make decisions now about the care I want in my later life.
- I will die free from pain, fear and with dignity, cared for by people who are trained and supported in high-quality palliative care.

2. I know that services are designed around me and my needs

I feel supported and understood by my general practitioner (GP) and get a physical check-up regularly without asking for it.

There are a range of services that support me with any aspect of daily living and enable me to stay at home and in my community, enjoying the best quality of life for as long as possible.

I am treated with dignity and respect whenever I need support from services.

I only go into hospital when I need to and when I get there staff understand how I can receive the best treatment so that I can leave as soon as possible.

Care home staff understand a lot about me and my disability and know what helps me cope and enjoy the best quality of life every day.

My carer can access respite care if and when needed, along with other services that can help support them in their role.

3. I have support that helps me live my life

- I can choose what support suits me best, so that I don't feel a burden.
- I can access a wide range of options and opportunities for support that suits me and my needs.
- I know how to get this support and I am confident it will help me.
- I have information and support and I can have fun with a network of others, including people in a position similar to mine.
- My carer also has a support network that suits their own needs.

4. I have the knowledge and know-how to get what I need

- It's not a problem getting information and advice, including information about the range of benefits I can access to help me afford and cope with living at home.
- I know where I can get the information I need when I need it, and I can digest and re-digest it in a way that suits me.
- I have enough information and advice to make decisions about managing, now and in the future, as my dementia progresses.
- My carer has access to further relevant information, and understands which benefits they are also entitled to.

5. I live in an enabling and supportive environment where I feel valued and understood

- I had a diagnosis very early on and, if I work, an understanding employer, which means I can still work and stay connected to people in my life.
- I am making a contribution, which makes me feel valued and valuable.
- My neighbours, friends, family and GP keep in touch and are pleased to see me.
- I am listened to and have my views considered, from the point I was first worried about my memory.
- The importance of helping me to sustain relationships with others is well recognised.
- If I develop behaviour that challenges others, people will take time to understand why I am acting in this way and help me to try to avoid it.
- My carer's role is respected and supported. They also feel valued and valuable, and neither of us feels alone.

6. I have a sense of belonging and of being a valued part of family, community and civic life

- I feel safe and supported in my home and in my community, which includes shops and pubs, sporting and cultural opportunities.
- Neither my family nor I feel ashamed or discriminated against because I have dementia. People with whom we come into contact are helpful and supportive.
- My carer and I continue to have the opportunity to develop new interests and new social networks.
- It is easy for me to continue to live in my own home, and my carer and I will both have the support needed for me to do this.

7. I know there is research going on that delivers a better life for me now and hope for the future

- I regularly read and hear about new developments in research.
- I am confident that there is an increasing investment in dementia research in the UK.
- I understand the growing evidence about prevention and risk reduction of dementia.
- As a person living with dementia, I am asked if I want to take part in suitable clinical trials or participate in research in other ways.
- I believe that research is key to improving the care I'm receiving now.
- I believe that more research will mean that my children and I can look forward to a range of treatments when I need it and there will be more treatments available for their generation.
- I know that with a diagnosis of dementia comes support to live well through assistive technologies as well as more traditional treatment types

At least as important as demographic growth is the changing expectations of a new generation of people with dementia, illustrated by the relatively modern demand for early diagnosis. The past decade has seen a dramatic shift from individuals 'turning a blind eye' to changes in their mental performance, to concern about whether these changes could represent the onset of dementia. Crucially, this concern is often accompanied by a wish to know if this is the case and asking for assessment. This new openness has revealed another fact; people over 50 now fear getting dementia more than they fear cancer.

Policy and politics

Dementia became a political issue in 2007 following publication of the report by the National Audit Office 'Improving services and support for people with dementia'. Included in the report was an economic analysis which showed that dementia costs the UK more than heart disease, stroke and cancer combined. Most of this cost was for care, either through Social Services or directly by patients and their families, rather than NHS costs. No longer was dementia a minor matter, it became the most expensive health condition the country faces.

One consequence was the National Dementia Strategy, which has guided changes in NHS care since, further clarified by the introduction of the National Institute for Health and Clinical Excellence (NICE) Dementia Standards. Currently, dementia has a high political profile, with the prime minister launching his own Dementia Challenge in 2012.

This book is written as a practical guide to the clinician who wishes to help the lives of those touched by dementia. Perhaps then we shall be guided by the voice of patients and the families who support them. The Dementia Action Alliance is made up of over 100 organisations. Through working with people with dementia and their families, the Dementia Action Alliance drew up the Dementia Declaration: A Call to Action, seven ambitious but achievable statements about how people can live well and what they would wish for from professionals – statements we should consider in our everyday clinical practice (Box 1).

CHAPTER 1

Dementia in the UK

Bernard Coope

Worcestershire Health and Care NHS Trust, Worcestershire, UK

OVERVIEW

- There are currently 8 00 000 people with dementia in the UK, and this number will rise to over a million by 2021.
- Dementia is the most expensive health care issue the country faces. The economic impact for 2012 was over £23 billion, more than heart disease, stroke and cancer combined.
- The syndrome of dementia consists of impairment of cognitive skills, resulting from disease of the brain, which is severe enough to impair daily functioning.
- There is more to dementia than memory impairment.
- Not all old people have dementia and not all people with dementia are old.

Introduction

Dementia is a clinical syndrome. This chapter examines the definition of dementia and explores a number of issues related to dementia as it is experienced in the UK.

Definition: The syndrome of dementia

The syndrome of dementia consists of three components:

1 impairment of cognitive skills,
2 resulting from disease of the brain,
3 which are severe enough to impair daily functioning.

It is worth taking time to look at the implications of this definition.

- **Dementia as a syndrome.** Central to the definition is a change in mental skills. To diagnose dementia, these changes need to be confidently identified, which usually means obtaining a careful history supported by an assessment of mental skills. Dementia relates to how well a person's brain is working rather than the presence of pathology, and can't be diagnosed from a brain scan any more than a plain X-ray of an arthritic joint can show pain. The diseases that cause dementia are covered in Chapter 2.

- **Cognitive functions are a diverse assortment of brain activity.** The term 'cognitive functions' covers memory encoding, long-term stores of knowledge, word finding, language comprehension, face or object recognition, planning and organising of activity and judgement. Different brain diseases lead to different patterns of cognitive change. There is more to dementia than memory impairment.

- **To diagnose dementia, there must be good reason to suspect disease of the brain.** Brain imaging may help, but in practice, brain disease is usually inferred from change in mental skill.

- **It is quite possible to have brain pathology without dementia.** As imaging techniques develop, it may soon be common to diagnose Alzheimer's disease years before any symptoms have developed. Vascular changes on imaging are very common and on their own don't mean vascular dementia.

- **Impairment of daily functioning is an important but imprecise term.** Very minor changes in mental skills are not usually referred to as dementia, although there may be a difference of opinion between patient, carer and clinician about when the change of functioning has occurred. For those with some detectable changes in mental function that are not impacting on daily functioning, the term *mild cognitive impairment* (MCI) is sometimes used.

- When discussing dementia, we should be careful not to use syndrome and pathology as interchangeable concepts.

Terminology

In the 1970s, the late Geriatrician Bernard Isaacs encouraged the use of the term 'chronic brain failure' as an alternative to dementia. The aim was to emphasise organ failure and to bring the definition in line with other commonly used terms, such as heart failure. 'Acute brain failure' represented delirium. Ultimately, the term was dropped as it had too many negative connotations, but the principle is worth reflecting on. Dementia is what we experience when changes in brain function impact on day to day life.

The National Audit Office in its groundbreaking report 'Improving Services and Support for People with Dementia' took a more blunt approach and chose the simple term 'progressive and terminal brain disease'. Whilst this may not respect the syndrome/pathology distinction, it had the merit of communicating the seriousness of dementia to a wide range of opinion formers and politicians.

ABC of Dementia, First Edition. Edited by Bernard Coope and Felicity Richards.
© 2014 John Wiley & Sons, Ltd. Published 2014 by John Wiley & Sons, Ltd.

Prevalence and demography

The Alzheimer's Society collated the following facts about dementia in 2012.

- There are currently 8 00 000 people with dementia in the UK.
- There are over 17 000 younger people with dementia in the UK.
- There are over 11 500 people with dementia from black and minority ethnic groups in the UK.
- There will be over a million people with dementia by 2021.
- Two-thirds of people with dementia are women.
- There are 6 70 000 carers of people with dementia in the UK.
- Family carers of people with dementia save the UK over £8 billion a year.
- Eighty percent of people living in care homes have a form of dementia or severe memory problems.
- Two-thirds of people with dementia live in the community while one-third live in a care home.
- Only 44% of people with dementia in England, Wales and Northern Ireland receive a diagnosis.

Economic impact

Until the National Audit Office published its report on dementia in 2007, dementia had never been considered a priority. It was the impact of dementia on the UK highlighted in this report that brought about a new political will to address the condition. The report detailed the real situation about dementia – not only how much the NHS and Social Services were spending on dementia but also what individuals spent on their own care and how much lost earnings could be attributed to carers taking time off work to provide care. The answer was a little over £17 billion.

The significance of this sum was that if other conditions underwent the same analysis, dementia cost the UK more than heart disease, stroke and cancer combined. Dementia is the most expensive health care issue the country faces, and it will continue on an upward trajectory. The economic impact for 2012 was over £23 billion.

Who has dementia?

The diseases that cause dementia get commoner as age advances, so the majority of those living with dementia are over 80. But not all old people have dementia and not all people with dementia are old. Dementia can occur in people under 65, when specialist skills are needed to address the complexities of diagnostic diversity, complex personal and family responses and age-related issues such as employment. The needs of younger people and their families are examined in Chapter 9.

As men tend to die younger than women, two-thirds of those with dementia are women. Age discrimination is gender discrimination! This can mean that care settings for people with dementia may have a greater proportion of woman – both residents and staff. Male residents may feel less comfortable in these environments, and are more likely to be perceived as challenging.

Dementia in learning disability is another area that requires specialist skills – from diagnosis, to helping that person live well. Dementia is more likely to develop at a young age in those with learning disability, especially Down's syndrome. The observation that people with Down's syndrome commonly developed dementia in their 40s indicated a link to chromosome 21 and ultimately to the discovery of the amyloid precursor gene.

Dementia is more likely to have a younger onset in black or ethnic minority groups, but these groups are underrepresented in services for dementia. Services need to take active steps to make sure that they reach out to minority communities and tackle barriers in assessment and support. The technical aspects of making a diagnosis have to take into account language, with testing being carried out in the person's preferred language where possible. Consideration needs to be given to educational background and also the cultural preconceptions embedded in many cognitive tests. Even a simple question like 'What is the season?' may be influenced by where an individual is from.

The Diversity of dementia

It is common for professionals to classify dementia into three stages of severity; mild, moderate and severe. However, it may be better to think of dementia as a journey a person is moving along, rather than a spectrum of disease severity – from what that individual previously considered as 'normal', through noticeable changes in mental skills that become consistent and then clear enough to warrant the use of the term dementia. As the person moves through the different stages of the condition, there is loss of mental skills. Other features may come and go, and quality of life is not closely linked to dementia severity. As an incurable condition, the person's journey will end in death resulting from dementia or other causes.

The journey of dementia is rarely made alone. Usually, close family support the person with dementia and inevitably their lives are also altered by it. Relatives start to be referred to as 'carers', although many are unhappy with that description. Carers' research commonly states the negatives of this role, such as burden, strain and stress, but there are also the positives. It is more useful to think about how the presence of dementia in a family changes relationships and how dementia is experienced in its entirety. This intricate interplay is addressed in detail in Chapter 6.

The changing journey

Loss of cognitive skills is the core feature of the dementia syndrome, but there is much more to it. A range of non-cognitive features can be experienced.

Psychosis

The presence of delusions (fixed, false beliefs) and hallucinations (perceptions without a corresponding object) are common at some point in dementia, although these experiences may be transient. Complex visual hallucinations are a core feature of dementia with Lewy body disease. Such features sometimes have little impact on the person with dementia, and have even been known to be enjoyable; however, they can also be extremely distressing and the cause of risky or aggressive behaviour. A person with dementia who believes that the spouse is an imposter may become understandably angry or violent towards them. Seeing dismembered bodies or snakes in the house can be frightening and lead a person to run out of the home. No longer believing your home is your own can be upsetting.

Affective disturbance

Depression commonly accompanies dementia, and again may be transient. The cause may be multifactorial, from the subjective experience of finding the world a bewildering place, having insight into their loss, the behaviour of others or directly due to brain disease. Depression is especially common in care home residents. It is usual to use antidepressant therapy, although there is little supportive evidence for this. Strategies aimed at improving quality of life through person-centred care and meaningful activity may be more productive.

Behavioural change

Behaviour that is out of character or challenging to others is distressing to loved ones and can be a major issue for those providing care. It is important not to see it as a symptom of dementia, although clearly the dementia is influencing it. Anger or shouting may arise from boredom, or pain. Behaviour is a communication and we should ask ourselves what is being communicated. The agitated woman looking for her mother can easily be seen as just forgetful and mistaken, or instead can be thought of as expressing the need for comfort and familiar attachment, leading to attempts to meet that need. The issue of behaviour that challenges is explored in Chapter 8.

Attachment

The word *attachment* appears repeatedly in this book. The concept was developed by John Bowlby and describes the nature of important and strong relationships. We have an evolved predisposition to form strong social bonds and the nature of our pattern of attachment forming is shaped by experiences early in life. The need for attachment never goes and is a healthy part of adult life. Even those with severe dementia will have a need for attachment, although the expression of this need may not be obvious, for example, searching for a long-lost mother when anxious. Understanding the person and the individual pattern of relationships, in the past and present, is a crucial component of person-centred care.

Physical disability and death

The brain diseases that cause dementias are commoner in older people, and so frequently accompany other health concerns that may be life-limiting. If this is not the case, dementias will become life-limiting in their own right. Loss of mobility and poor swallowing result in a higher risk of infections. It is probably better to view this as the late stages of severe brain disease, rather than simply an acute illness. Good palliative care at the end of life starts with recognising the impact of severe dementia. Early diagnosis offers a chance for people to make their future wishes known and plan appropriate care and place of death.

But the journey for the family goes on after death. Research shows that bereavement experiences may be longer and deeper after a death from dementia. Indeed, grief reactions occur in relatives long before the person with dementia has died. Good care at the end of life, working with families and bereavement support can help this. Chapter 13 addresses this important and often neglected area.

Who can help?

Who can help?

The person with dementia
Family and friends
Primary care
Social care and housing
Acute hospitals
Specialist mental health teams
Voluntary sector

The person with dementia. Not the most obvious start, as people with dementia are often thought of as passive recipients of care. An early diagnosis gives the person with early dementia time to plan life and express wishes for the future.

Family and friends. People who provide the bulk of dementia care in the UK. Professionals could see their role as helping families to understand dementia and how to provide care.

Primary care. General practitioners (GPs) and other primary care staff are well placed to help the person with dementia live well. There may already be an established relationship with a GP, who may also know other members of the family and will have a much broader view of the entirety of the person's health than specialists. Dementia in primary care is the subject of Chapter 10.

Social care. People with dementia and their carers are entitled to a benefits check – for attendance allowance and carers' allowance. A carers' assessment should be offered to all informal carers. Formal care arrangements may enable a person to remain at home with additional support for many years, for example, offering help with personal care, nutrition and medication compliance. Community social workers can help guide people with dementia and their families in this area. Services like direct payments are particularly useful in early dementia, to allow an individual with dementia plan the required support. Respite placements are also an option to give informal carers a break from this role.

Assistive technology

Recent years have seen a growth in technological ways to support a person with dementia maintain independence and stay safe. A Global Positioning System (GPS) locator may help give greater confidence to someone who enjoys a daily walk but might get lost. Automated tablet dispensers with alarms can help in compliance. It is a rapidly changing field that can support but not replace the presence of a carer.

Care homes. It may well be that the needs of a person with dementia change to a level where long-term placement has to be arranged. A third of people with dementia live in a residential or nursing home. Developing skills in dementia care takes time and effort but it is important for staff and residents alike.

Acute hospitals. People with dementia find acute hospitals challenging places to be in, and hospitals can find people with dementia challenging, too. These issues and solutions are discussed in Chapter 11.

Specialist mental health teams. Older adult Community Mental Health Teams (CMHTs) are multidisciplinary teams that work with people with dementia and others with poor mental health. They will usually include psychiatrists, community psychiatric nurses (CPNs), occupational therapists and social workers. They will usually work with people at greatest need (risk, challenging behaviour, carer breakdown) and are not in a position to follow up people indefinitely. They offer 'stepping stones' of specialist care along the journey of dementia. Memory Clinics or Early Intervention Dementia Services can deal with diagnostic assessments and drug treatments. Admiral nurses, specialists in supporting families affected by dementia, sometimes work alongside CMHTs.

Voluntary sector. Organisations like the Alzheimer's Society and Age UK can provide a wealth of information, through excellent Internet-based sites to more direct and personalised provision. In some parts of the country, these services are commissioned to provide dementia advisors, people who can be approached for advice and signposting. Dementia Cafés are regular gatherings for people with dementia and their families for peer support and they make a very positive contribution to helping those with dementia live well.

Conclusion

For the first time, dementia is being recognised as an important issue faced by the country and one that challenges the NHS in many ways. Between the old, futile pessimism of 'There's no point in thinking about dementia as nothing can be done' and the new oversimplified optimism of 'We can prevent dementia or stop it getting worse so everyone should have an early diagnosis', there lies a wealth of real opportunities to help the lives of those living with dementia. The National Institute of Clinical Excellence has published 10 quality standards for the NHS that encapsulate this.

NICE	10 quality standards
Statement 1	People with dementia receive care from staff appropriately trained in dementia care.
Statement 2	People with suspected dementia are referred to a memory assessment service specialising in the diagnosis and initial management of dementia.
Statement 3	People newly diagnosed with dementia and/or their carers receive written and verbal information about their condition, treatment and the support options in their local area.
Statement 4	People with dementia have an assessment and an ongoing personalised care plan, agreed across health and social care, that identifies a named care coordinator and addresses their individual needs.
Statement 5	People with dementia, while they have capacity, have the opportunity to discuss and make decisions, together with their carer/s, about the use of advance statements or advance decisions to refuse treatment, lasting power of attorney and preferred priorities of care.
Statement 6	Carers of people with dementia are offered an assessment of emotional, psychological and social needs and, if accepted, receive tailored interventions identified by a care plan to address those needs.
Statement 7	People with dementia who develop non-cognitive symptoms that cause them significant distress, or who develop behaviour that challenges, are offered an assessment at an early opportunity to establish generating and aggravating factors. Interventions to improve such behaviour or distress should be recorded in their care plan.
Statement 8	People with suspected or known dementia using acute and general hospital inpatient services or emergency departments have access to a liaison service that specialises in the diagnosis and management of dementia and older people's mental health.
Statement 9	People in the later stages of dementia are assessed by primary care teams to identify and plan their palliative care needs.
Statement 10	Carers of people with dementia have access to a comprehensive range of respite/short-break services that meet the needs of both the carer and the person with dementia.

Further reading

Alzheimer's Society, *Dementia 2012, A National Challenge*. 2012. www.alzheimers.org.uk

National Audit Office, *Improving Services and Support for People with Dementia*. 2007. www.nao.org.uk

National Institute for Health and Care Excellence. *Dementia Quality Standards*. 2010. www.nice.org.uk

CHAPTER 2

Causes of Dementia

Georgios Theodoulou

Worcestershire Care and Health NHS Trust, Worcestershire

OVERVIEW

- Different diseases of the brain cause different changes in mental function.
- Alzheimer's disease (AD) is still the leading cause of dementia in the UK.
- There is an interplay between the environment and genes in the development of dementia.
- Vascular risk factors are associated with a higher risk for dementias including AD.

Introduction

The varied phenotypes of dementia reflect a multitude of causes (see Table 2.1). A better understanding of these aids an accurate diagnosis, which, in turn, should help the person with dementia and their carer(s) access the appropriate support and available pharmacological treatments where indicated. Moreover, a better understanding of the pathology of the different phenotypes will hopefully lead to novel and more successful psychosocial and pharmacological treatments. The main causes of dementia are listed in Table 2.2 and are discussed in detail in this chapter. The less common causes of dementia syndromes are also listed (see Table 2.3).

Alzheimer's disease (AD)

There are three main AD phenotypes:

1 Typical AD
2 Posterior Cortical Atrophy (PCA)
3 Logopenic Aphasia (LA)

Clinical features

In each case, the cellular pathology is similar but the distribution of the pathology leads to the characteristic clinical presentations.

ABC of Dementia, First Edition. Edited by Bernard Coope and Felicity Richards.
© 2014 John Wiley & Sons, Ltd. Published 2014 by John Wiley & Sons, Ltd.

Typical AD

Typical AD mostly affects older people, especially those in their late 70s–80s. It presents with insidiously worsening memory, most obviously in new learning but also in recall of previously learnt memories. Attention and concentration are relatively well preserved.

This amnesic presentation relates to the predilection of Alzheimer's pathology for medial structures of the hippocampus and cingulate gyrus.

Over a number of years, the disease process spreads out across the cortex to affect the temporal, parietal and frontal lobes, with relative sparing of the occipital lobes. Subtle language impairments commonly occur with amnesia, and frontal involvement leads to poor planning and organising skills.

Table 2.1 Classification of primary neurodegenerative pathologies causing dementias.

Tauopathies	Progressive Supranuclear Palsy, Corticobasilar Degeneration, PiD and FTDP17 (?AD)
α-synucleinopathies	Parkinson's disease dementia/dementia with Lewy bodies
Amyloidopathies	Alzheimer's disease
Prion disease	Creutzfeldt–Jakob disease (CJD)
Polyglutamine disease	Huntington's disease

Table 2.2 Main causes of dementia (relative proportion in percentage).

Alzheimer's disease (62%)
Cerebrovascular disease (17%)
Mixed Alzheimer and cerebrovascular disease (10%)
Dementia with Lewy bodies/Parkinson's disease (6%)
Frontotemporal dementia syndromes (2%)
Less common causes of dementia syndromes
Alcohol
Multiple sclerosis
Normal pressure hydrocephalus
Paraneoplastic/autoimmune
Huntington's disease
Wilson's disease
CJD
HIV/AIDS dementia complex
Metachromic leucodystrophy
Space-occupying lesions

With disease progression, language impairments become more obvious, with anomia and grammatical changes. In severe disease, an individual's basic understanding and communication becomes severely affected and greater physical disability occurs, with deteriorating mobility, swallowing difficulties and incontinence. The onset of these features makes the individual vulnerable to life-limiting infections and poor nutrition (see Chapter 13).

Posterior cortical atrophy

In PCA, the AD pathology mostly affects occipital areas, leading to early change in visuospatial skills. Visual recognition of objects is affected as is the location of objects in space. The can be thought of as the 'what' and the 'where' of spatial thinking. It is not just visual skills but the person's ability to think in three dimensions that changes; this can lead to early loss of practical skills such as dressing.

The triad of Balint's syndrome of oculomotor apraxia (difficulty fixing the gaze on an object), optic ataxia (difficulty guiding the hand to an object by vision) and simultanagnosia (difficulty perceiving multiple objects in the visual field) is sometimes elicited.

In early stages, other areas of the brain are spared, so memory, language and frontal functions are less affected. Patients often have clear recall of their difficulties and can articulate them clearly. Paradoxically, this means that they may not be taken seriously, a problem compounded by often good performances on simple cognitive assessments. PCA is found in a younger age group than typical AD.

Logopenic aphasia

LA is a primary progressive aphasia, manifesting as prominent early changes in fluent speech production. It resembles progressive non-fluent aphasia (PNFA, a type of frontotemporal dementia) but is usually not a pure language disorder as it is often accompanied with deficits in visual memory and visuospatial skills. The absence of speech apraxia (problems repeating polysyllabic words) helps distinguish it from PNFA. As the condition progresses, it starts to resemble typical AD.

Pathology of Alzheimer's disease

All three subtypes have the pathological hallmarks of beta amyloid ($A\beta$)-containing senile plaques and highly phosphorylated tau-protein-containing neurofibrillary tangles (NFTs), which, to some extent, also occur in healthy brains – the 'amyloid cascade hypothesis' (see Box 2.1). The pathology leads to disruption in acetylcholine neuronal systems projecting from the nucleus basalis of Meynert, the 'cholinergic hypothesis'. Serotenergic and noradrenergic projections are also affected to a lesser degree.

Box 2.1 **Breakdown of the amyloid cascade hypothesis**

– Amyloid precursor protein (APP) is coded on chromosome 21 and is sequentially cleaved by alpha, beta and gamma secretase enzymes into $A\beta$.
– $A\beta$ varies in length between 37 and 42 amino acids. Senile plaques in AD are predominantly composed of $A\beta$ of 42 amino acid length ($A\beta$ 42). Where there is a disproportionate amount of gamma secretase activity, a greater proportion of $A\beta42$ is produced (the predominant cleavage pathway is that of the alpha secretase (95%) leading to non-amyloidgenic pathways).
– Gamma sectretase has two identified mutations – Presenilin 1 and Presenilin 2 and accounts for 5% of familial Alzheimer's disease (FAD).
– The modified amyloid cascade hypothesis states that abnormal amyloid deposition precedes the formation of NFTs, although how one leads onto another is not clear. Tau protein is important for microtubule function and so dysfunction here as in NFT formation will disrupt cell structure leading to cell death.

Vascular dementia (VaD)

Clinical features

The functioning of the brain can be impaired by ischaemia. The clinical presentation of vascular dementia is diverse, with variations in time course and changes in mental skills. The stepwise deterioration with plateaus classically described in VaD is perhaps overstated, reflecting the uncommon presentation of pure multiple strategic infarcts.

Areas of poor brain function due to cortical ischaemia can produce focal cognitive change (e.g. dysphasia or impaired facial recognition), yet the same individual may have some brain functions that are unaffected.

An insidious onset of patchy episodic memory impairment similar to an AD presentation is common in VaD. Executive and visuospatial difficulties, inattention, mental slowing and apathy tend to be more common earlier in its course compared to AD as are emotional changes of depression or labile emotions. Daily fluctuations and nocturnal worsening are common (cf. AD). Psychotic phenomena occur in VaD and may mimic symptoms associated with Lewy body disease.

Sub-cortical impairment may cause less obvious changes in concentration or motivation, which can be both disabling and challenging to carers.

Pathology of VaD

Ischaemic damage to the brain can occur through microangiopathy (diffuse small vessel disease), strategic infarction or multiple lacunar infarction. Vasculitis may also cause ischaemic damage. The greater the cell volume loss, the greater the impairment, although the site of damage is also relevant, for example, bilateral thalamic infarcts may produce profound amnesia. A dominantly inherited form of diffuse white matter disease is known as cerebral autosomal dominant arteriopathy, with subcortical infarcts and leukoencephalopathy (CADASIL).

There will usually be evidence of vascular risk factors and vascular disease elsewhere.

Mixed AD and VaD

Clinical features and pathology as for VaD and AD

The coexistence of both Alzheimer's pathology and vascular disease may produce dementia even where the presence of either pathology alone would not be sufficient to produce a dementia syndrome. Both conditions are common but occur together more commonly by chance alone. This is probably because they share some risk factors, for example, diabetes and the ApoE genotype.

Dementia with Lewy bodies (DLB)/Parkinson disease dementia (PDD)

Clinical features

Dementia with Lewy bodies and Parkinson's disease dementia are clinical presentations of Lewy body pathology in the brain. Both conditions are considered to be on the same spectrum of disorder.

In DLB, the initial presentation is of cognitive change, commonly involving visuospatial skills with relatively intact memory. Other features accompany the deficits in mental skills, including visual hallucinations, marked fluctuations in attention and consciousness, extrapyramidal signs, falls, rapid eye movement (REM) sleep behaviour disorder and neuroleptic sensitivity. The sensitivity to neuroleptic or antipsychotic drugs is severe and can be life-threatening. These changes may mimic acute delirium, and the diagnosis can depend on a detailed longitudinal history from an informant.

In DLB, the parkinsonian features may be subtle, a lack of facial expression, bradykinesia and rigidity, or monotonous voice that can easily be mistaken for depression. The gait may be shuffling with loss of arm swing, but tremor is less common.

Up to 80% of those with established Parkinson's disease may go on to develop dementia and this is usually referred to as Parkinson's disease dementia, with a presentation very similar to DLB.

Pathology of DLB/PDD

Lewy bodies are inclusions within the cytoplasm of neurons composed of α-synuclein as well as other proteins including ubiquitin and neurofilament protein. Alzheimer's pathology also coexists in DLB. The deficit of acetylcholine function is greater than in AD and patients may gain symptomatic benefit from treatment with acetylcholinesterase inhibitors.

Frontotemporal dementias (FTDs)

The frontotemporal dementias (FTDs) are a heterogeneous group of dementias caused by an increasing number of individually identified pathologies. Broadly, three phenotypes have been described to date:

1 Behavioural variant (bv-FTD)
2 Semantic dementia (SD)
3 Progressive non-fluent aphasia (PNFA)

Clinical features
Behavioural variant

Bv-FTD presents with changes in personality and behaviour. Loss of social awareness, disinhibition, impulsiveness, apathy, mental rigidity, new obsessions and changes in eating habits, often with a predilection for sweet foods and personal neglect, are common features.

Semantic dementia

SD presents with loss of memory for the meaning of words, that is, semantic knowledge. Speech production reduces and is simplified, for example, using categorical words like 'animal' or 'thing' rather than more specific terms. There is an associated loss of knowledge of objects that goes beyond word use. Memory and orientation are not usually affected early on. More typical features of the bv-FTD phenotype will develop later in the course.

Progressive Non-Fluent Aphasia

PNFA presents with a severe disruption of speech output, with grammatical and phonological errors. The speech is hesitant, and produced with great effort. Mild executive dysfunction is also common, but memory and attention remain relatively intact early on. Symptoms can often cause great distress. The condition can seem relatively stable and unchanging for many years.

Pathology of FTD

A number of different pathologies are associated with FTD. Approximately 50% of FTD is associated with tau pathology. Frontotemporal dementia syndromes can be associated with other conditions. Progressive supranuclear palsy (PSP), corticobasal degeneration (CBD), FTD with parkinsonism linked to chromosome 17 (FTDP-17) and motor neuron disease (MND) can all independently be associated with FTD.

Normal pressure hydrocephalus

Clinical features

Normal pressure hydrocephalus usually presents with a triad of mild cognitive difficulties, a wide-based gait and urinary incontinence. Many of these symptoms are common in the elderly, and the latter two are usually features of the middle to later stages of other dementias.

Pathology of NPH

NPH is somewhat of a misnomer, as on average the intracranial pressure is a little above normal limits with frequent additional pulses known as 'B' waves. The underlying mechanism of how this translates into cerebral dysfunction and damage is not yet elucidated but is thought to, at least in part, lead to chronic mild periventricular white matter ischaemia.

Risks and protective factors in the aetiology of dementia

Aetiological studies in dementia have to date mainly focused on the dementia syndrome in general or specifically on Alzheimer's dementia. Studies on the aetiology of other dementias are less common. By identifying individual factors that protect against or increase the risk of dementia we may be able to develop primary prevention interventions.

Table 2.3 Other types of dementia.

Huntington's disease

Autosomal-dominant degenerative disease characterised by progressive psychiatric and movement disorder followed by dementia. A triplet repeat disorder with a mutation in the Huntington gene on chromosome 4, which causes an enlarged polyglutamine portion to be added to the Huntington protein. Mutated forms aggregate within neurons, causing cell death.

Creutzfelt–Jacob disease (CJD)/prion disease

Rapidly progressive dementia associated with epilepsy. Pathogenic process involves conversion of a normal cell surface protein termed *cellular prion protein* into an abnormally folded and protease-resistant isoform. A small minority (15%) are found to be caused by a mutation in the prion protein gene but the majority are sporadic, classically caused by CJD.

Multiple sclerosis

Chronic disease of the central nervous system (CNS). Involves inflammatory, demyelinating and neurodegenerative processes. Primary, secondary and relapsing/remitting forms. Dementia may form part of the neuropsychiatric presentation of multiple sclerosis (MS), and on rare occasions be the only manifestation of MS. Pattern and severity of cognitive deficits not correlated with either disease duration or physical disability.

Limbic encephalitis

Encompasses a range of inflammatory conditions selectively affecting the limbic system (amygdala, hippocampus, hypothalamus, insular cortex and cingulate cortex). These can present with a relatively rapid-onset dementia and/or other neuropsychiatric signs and symptoms. Originally thought to only be associated with an autoimmune response to cancer or infection elsewhere in the body, it is now recognised to be related to autoantibodies to voltage-gated potassium channels (VGKCs) and N-methyl d-aspartate (NMDA) receptors. Potentially treatable with plasma exchange.

HIV/AIDS dementia complex

Feature of advanced HIV 1 disease progression, rare with early antiretroviral use. HIV 1 is neurotropic but necessarily pathogenic in the CNS; nevertheless, it is theorised that in some cases infection leads to an inflammatory cascade, leading in turn to cell death through cytokine.

Metachromic leucodystrophy

One of a group of genetic lipid storage disorders. Thought to be caused by arylsulfatase A enzyme deficiency. This in turn impairs growth or development of the myelin sheath. Adult form presents with neurological signs as well as dementia.

Space-occupying lesions (SOLs) – tumours/subdural haematomas

Account for 3% of all cases of dementia. SOLs in certain parts of the brain may increase intracranial pressure, causing dementia. A classic tumour lesion producing signs of dementia is frontal lobe meningioma.

Alcohol

Alcohol has direct neurotoxic effects on brain cells with chronic excessive exposure.

(i) Age

Dementia increases in prevalence and incidence with increasing age.

(ii) Gender

Approximately two-thirds of people with dementia are women.

(iii) Education

Education may enhance neurological reserve, so greater pathology is required to cause cognitive deficits as well as there being a greater capacity to compensate for the pathology.

(iv) Genetics

The APOE ϵ4 allele is an established risk factor for developing dementia. It is present in about 25–30% of the population and in about 40% of all people with late-onset Alzheimer's. Although the APOE ϵ4 allele is a susceptibility gene, homozygotic carriers do not necessarily develop dementia. There is tentative evidence of an interaction between the APOE ϵ4 allele with stroke, hypertension and alcohol in specifically increasing the risk of dementia. The APOE ϵ2 allele appears to protect against the development of dementia. The APOE gene on chromosome 19 plays a part in lipid metabolism in neuronal health.

There are rare families where young-onset AD has a familial dominantly inherited pattern involving the presenilin 1 (Ch14) and 2 (Ch1) genes encoding for the splicing of APP. In Down's syndrome (trisomy 21), there is an association with excess APP production and abnormal secretase activity both coded for on Ch21 leading to AD.

It is increasingly recognised that of the heritable FTDs, a large minority are associated with abnormalities on Ch17 where tau protein metabolism is coded for (FTDP-17).

(v) Smoking

More recent studies have shown that smoking increases the risk of developing dementia, although it is debatable if nicotine alone may have a protective effect for some dementias.

(vi) Alcohol

There is a clear relationship with heavy alcohol use leading to an increased risk of dementia. There are several mechanisms including the direct toxic effects of alcohol on the brain as well as the increased prevalence of cerebrovascular disease in those who drink excessive alcohol. Indirect effects include the greater prevalence of head injury and thiamine deficiency, which are both risk factors for cognitive impairment in heavy alcohol users.

(vii) Cholesterol

The evidence at present is equivocal as to the influence cholesterol has on the development of dementia. The use of statins has not been found to reduce the incidence of dementia.

(viii) Blood pressure

Mid-life hypertension is associated with both VaD and AD later in life. In those over 75 years of age, it is hypotension that appears to be the main risk factor, and indeed by raising the blood pressure the brain appears to benefit for the increased perfusion.

(ix) Diabetes mellitus

DM increases the risk of most degenerative dementias. In the very old, there is an increased risk of developing dementia with impaired glucose tolerance even in the absence of frank DM. Putative theories include the effects of long-term hyperglycaemia causing neurodegeneration as well as the effects of raised insulin levels in the brain for Type II DM.

(x) Heart disease

Heart disease is associated with an increased risk of both VaD and Alzheimer's especially in those with combined peripheral vascular disease. Atrial fibrillation and congestive cardiac failure also contribute to the risk of developing dementia and may be independent risk factors.

(xi) Body mass index

During mid-life, a high BMI is associated with an increased risk of dementia. In later life, a relatively steady drop in BMI over a few years may herald the beginnings of dementia.

(xii) Diet

Evidence that specific components of a healthy diet affecting the risk of developing dementia is lacking. Antioxidant vitamins A, E and C are unlikely to have long-term neuroprotective effects. There is a relationship between vitamin B12, folic acid and homocysteine in that the first two reduce the serum levels of the latter. A raised serum homocysteine level is a known risk factor for heart and cerebrovascular disease, which, in turn, increases the risk of dementia. The OPTIMA (Oxford Project to Investigate Memory and Aging) study found that blood homocysteine levels were significantly higher, and blood folic acid and vitamin B12 levels significantly lower, in patients with confirmed Alzheimer's disease.

Saturated fats, in general, are associated with an increased risk of vascular disease, raising the possibility that they increase the risk of dementia. Fish polyunsaturated fats may have a more direct relationship with reducing dementia risk, although the studies to date are equivocal.

(xiii) Social, leisure and physical activity

Maintaining an active, enjoyable and mentally stimulating lifestyle, particularly in mid to later life is associated with reducing the risk of developing dementia.

Table 2.4 Possible primary prevention.

Control for vascular risk factors
Eat a healthy and balanced diet
Drink alcohol in small quantities
Keep physically active
Maintain a good social network
Continue hobbies and interests into later life
Keep enjoying life

(xiv) Other factors

Hormone replacement therapy (HRT) and non-steroidal anti-inflammatory drugs (NSAIDs) are not evidenced as reducing dementia risk. Traumatic brain injury, depression and later life delirium may be associated with an increased risk of dementia.

Primary prevention

To date, there is no evidence to show that dementia can be prevented or delayed, even in the brains of those at higher risk. Nevertheless, taking into account the available evidence on risk factors for developing dementia, sensible advice is highlighted in Table 2.4.

Further reading

Hodges J. *Frontotemporal Dementia Syndromes*. Cambridge University Press, 2007.

Dickson D, Weller RO (eds). *Neurodegeneration: The Molecular Pathology of Dementia and Movement Disorder*. Wiley-Blackwell, 2011.

Jacoby R, Oppenheimer C, Dening T and Thomas A. *Oxford Textbook of Old Age Psychiatry*. Oxford University Press, 2008.

CHAPTER 3

Assessment

Bernard Coope and Felicity A. Richards

Worcestershire Health and Care NHS Trust, Worcestershire, UK

OVERVIEW

- Making a diagnosis of dementia is essentially a clinical decision reached by assimilating the patient's history, cognitive assessment and imaging.
- There is more to assessment than making a diagnosis. What else needs to be addressed to help the person with dementia?
- Always consider a patient's wishes around assessment, including their wish to know, or not know the potential diagnosis.
- Cognitive testing varies greatly, and testing should be guided by the clinical history of change.
- A diagnosis is never more than the best explanation for the findings, not absolute fact.

Introduction

In this chapter, the assessment of dementia is addressed with the use of three questions:

1 **Why**? What is the purpose of the assessment?
2 **What** exactly are you assessing?
3 **How** do you go about gathering the information you need in order to make a diagnosis?

Why?

Before commencing an assessment with a person with possible dementia, it is important to consider the question of why you are doing it. It is worth stating the obvious here; the reason we assess an individual is in the hope that it will be helpful to that person in some way. This may be directly helpful, that is, clarifying the diagnosis to a person with concerns about memory. Or benefits of an assessment may be more indirect; it can be valuable to professionals or family members to know about the diagnosis in order to better understand the condition or make the best plans for care.

In the past decade, society has moved away from the belief that a diagnosis of dementia is unimportant, to one where making a diagnosis is viewed unquestioningly as a good thing. This complete

about turn has led to considerable pressure to increase diagnosis rates as though this is an end in itself. It is not.

We should also be mindful that like any health care intervention, dementia assessment has the potential to do harm. Proper consideration should also be given to informed consent. In the case of an individual lacking the mental capacity to consent, the assessment must be in that person's best interests.

What?

A health assessment may have many different components (see Box 3.1). We may be interested in finding out if the person has a clinical syndrome of dementia. If so, we may want more detail, for example, how severe is it, or what is the likely disease process that is causing the dementia? From a practical point of view, it may be valuable to understand the pattern of cognitive losses and preserved skills, to aid understanding and care planning.

If we are to help a person live well with dementia, we may be more interested in the sources of support, who the carers are and how the carers/family may be feeling. Is there any risk arising from the dementia? If there are important decisions to be made, does the person have the capacity to make these decisions?

Box 3.1 Different reasons to assess for presence of a dementia

Is dementia present?
What brain disease is present?
What care needs are there?
Is there risk?
Does the person have the mental capacity to make a decision at this time?
How is the carer and what would help them?

How?

The exact nature of the assessment will be determined by its purpose. If the aim is to make a diagnosis of dementia and also to clarify the underlying brain disease, the assessment is essentially a three-piece jigsaw puzzle consisting of a clinical history, cognitive testing and imaging. Of these, the history is by far the most

---

important, with cognitive testing and imaging providing useful supportive information (Box 3.2).

> Box 3.2 **The assessment of dementia – A three-piece jigsaw**
>
> **1** Clinical history
> **2** Cognitive testing
> **3** Imaging

The story of change

A good description of change in mental skills is where assessment starts (see Box 3.3). The extent to which the person can contribute to the assessment process will depend on the severity or type of dementia. Most people with mild or moderate dementia will be able to give some subjective description of how they are.

Contrary to conventional teaching, most people with mild dementia are very aware of change in mental skills. It is also extremely important to gather this description of change from at least one other person who knows them well. This can be an uncomfortable situation, but it is usually best to hold the interview together rather than to talk secretively. Quite commonly, an informant will be more concerned about mental skills than the patient. Sometimes a person will seek help alone, saying that they don't want to worry their family, and in these cases dementia is less likely to be present.

> Box 3.3 **Points of diagnostic value**
>
> **Duration and change over time that may suggest likely pathological process**
>
> Sudden onset: suggests a vascular aetiology
> Gradual change over a few years: suggests degenerative disease
> Progressive change over days, weeks or months: very concerning, may indicate space-occupying lesion, subdural, delirium, and so on
> Past 20 years/all my life: unlikely to be degenerative condition such as dementia
>
> **What has changed?**
>
> Memory
> Language
> Visuospatial skills
> Judgement and personality

What has changed?

Memory

'My memory is dreadful, doctor' is not enough. This is a common subjective concern and can accompany depression, low self-esteem or a fear of getting dementia. Most changes in memory lead to impairment in storing new memories, sometimes inaccurately described as 'short-term memory'. Poor recall of old memories can also occur, as can a loss of general knowledge.

Ask for specific examples such as forgetting conversations or recent events. Repetitiveness usually accompanies forgetting, although it must be distinguished from the repetitiveness that may accompany depression, anxiety or obsessional thinking. Memory deficits will nearly always be more obvious to the informant.

Language

Changes in language skills are common and important to detect. In some dementia syndromes, they may be the major presenting feature and can cause great distress. Disturbance in language skills indicates dysfunction of the dominant (usually left) hemisphere.

Changes in language may be subtle. Problems with finding words (anomia) may be mistakenly described as 'forgetting' words. It may lead to breaks when speaking or the increasing use of paraphasias ('thingummy') or circumlocutions ('thing that tells you the time' for clock). Sometimes there may be word errors, the wrong word slipping out, either a similar sounding word 'parcark' for 'carpark' or a word from a similar semantic category. Other important language skill changes include changes in spelling, grammar or articulation of polysyllabic words (speech apraxia).

Visuospatial skills

Changes in the brain's ability to process visual information may have a big impact on daily living skills, for example, putting on clothes, navigating in familiar or unfamiliar places (topographical memory), putting things in the right place or recognising or using familiar objects.

These skills can involve the 'what' of visual information, leading to recognition errors, or the 'where', leading to difficulties in locating things, for example, reaching past objects. These changes suggest dysfunction of parietal or occipital lobes. Problems recognising faces (prosopagnosia) is associated with the inferior occipital lobe and fusiform gyrus and can occur independently of visuospatial deficits for other objects.

In the history, visuospatial difficulties will sometimes be talked about as a memory problem, that is, 'my father's forgotten how to use the cooker' 'my sister can't remember where the bathroom is', so it is important to elucidate the exact nature of these complaints.

Judgement and personality

Behaviour that appears out of character can sometimes be associated with organic brain disease, although it can also occur for many other reasons. It is associated with pathology in the frontal lobes. Loss of empathy is a core feature, with family members describing a loss of regard for the feelings of others.

Behaviour may become more socially inappropriate, sometimes including offensive or illegal activities such as shoplifting or sexual assault. Importantly, such acts are impulsive and don't show any advanced planning. Despite these changes, apathy and diminished motivation commonly accompany the clinical picture, which can help differentiate the state from hypomania.

Testing cognitive ability

Measurement of cognitive skills is an essential complement to the history. Formal testing must be guided by the information gathered in the history: both changes in mental skills and any other factor(s) that could confound the test score (see Box 3.4).

Box 3.4 Factors that alter cognitive test scores

High premorbid intellect
Low educational attainment, truanting, poor literacy
Low IQ, learning disability
Poor vision or hearing
Not carrying out test in first language
Motivation/cooperation/mood
Cultural differences

Cognitive tests vary depending on the purpose and also on the severity of dementia. Picking up possible signs of dementia to guide referral or hospital care can be achieved with a short test such as Abbreviated Mental Test Score (AMTS), General Practitioner Assessment of Cognition (GPCOG), or 6-Item Cognitive Impairment Test (6CIT). The more advanced the dementia, the more obvious the changes in cognitive skills tend to be; therefore, confirming the presence of severe dementia may only require some brief tests of memory and orientation.

To confidently diagnose early dementia will require more detailed testing. Sometimes it may be important to measure the severity of dementia for staging, measuring treatment response or research. For specialist memory assessment services, the Addenbrookes Cognitive Examination (ACE) is commonly used (see Box 3.5). Further, more detailed neuropsychometric testing may be required.

Cognitive testing needs to be carried out with skill and care. The same consideration needs to be given as would be given for a physical examination, in other words, explanation of the test and why it is being done, privacy and consent. The patient will usually need to be seated at a table, with no background noise and reading glasses or hearing aids available. The presence of family may be reassuring or distracting and embarrassing. Ask patients how they feel about others being present.

Box 3.5 Cognitive tests

Short tests for brief screening in the acute setting or primary care

AMT score. A 10-point test that can identify severe impairment of cognitive skills as found in a moderate/severe dementia or delirium.
Mini Mental State Examination (MMSE). Widely used test, 30 points. Use limited by authors retaining copyright.
Test Your Memory (TYM). A short, self-administered test developed for screening.
The Montreal Cognitive Assessment (MOCA). A 30-point test sensitive to mild cognitive changes and covering a range of cognitive functions.
General Practitioner test of cognitive function (GP COG). A brief test developed for use in primary care. Relatively unaffected by educational and cultural background. Includes a test for the person with concerns and a carer questionnaire.

6CIT. A brief test that takes 5 min to administer; validated in primary care.

Longer test for memory clinic/diagnosis

Addenbrookes Cognitive Assessment (ACE). A 100-point test, taking approximately 20 min to complete. Provides an overall score and subscores of different cognitive domains. Includes sections to detect non-Alzheimer's dementia.

Examples of detailed cognitive tests for specialist use or research.

Intelligence ((Verbal and Performance): WAIS-R Wechsler Adult Intelligence Scale
Repeatable Battery for the Assessment of Neuropsychological Status (RBANS)

Imaging

Where cognitive testing gives an indication of brain function, brain imaging gives an indication of its appearance. Imaging is currently recommended as one component of diagnostic assessment. It is important to recognise the limitation of imaging, and for both clinicians and patients not to overemphasise the importance of imaging in making a dementia diagnosis. Remember that with advancing age, brain scans appear increasingly abnormal. Atrophy and signs of vascular disease are almost invariable in a person over 70, regardless of cognitive function.

– Is there something that shouldn't be there?

  Subdural haematomas, tumours or normal pressure hydrocephalus can be identified on structural imaging.

– Is the brain different from expected?

  Localised atrophy may support a diagnosis, especially if it matches findings from history and testing. This can be valuable in Alzheimer's disease, frontotemporal dementia syndromes or posterior cortical atrophy, especially when investigating younger people where atrophy would be unexpected. Vascular changes can also be visualised, although the presence of vascular disease does not mean that this is the only pathology, and does not in itself diagnose dementia. Likewise, a scan can be normal in a patient with Alzheimer's disease.

Box 3.6 List of commonly used imaging techniques

Computerised tomography (CT)

Quick, available and well tolerated by the majority of patients. CT is suitable for excluding space-occupying lesions.

Magnetic resonance imaging (MRI)

This test is noisy, slow and confined, and therefore can be an uncomfortable for some older or impaired patients. Images show structures in higher resolution, detect vascular changes well and allows visualisation from different views. Coronal images may allow hippocampal atrophy in Alzheimer's disease to be seen.

Functional imaging

This is not currently recommended for routine clinical use, although it has value in research and may become more commonly used as part of diagnostic investigation.

The diagnosis

Making a diagnosis is essentially a clinical decision reached by assimilating the patient's history, cognitive assessment and imaging. The more these components marry up, the more confidence the clinician can feel about the diagnosis.

It can be helpful to think of the diagnosis in two stages:

1 Is there evidence of the dementia syndrome?
2 What is the likely disease process causing the dementia?

It is also important to remember that a diagnosis is never more than the best explanation for the findings, not absolute fact.

Finally, as with most areas of medicine, it is easier to say that enough evidence has been found to make a diagnosis than it is to say that there is nothing wrong with a patient. Patients looking for reassurance may find this inability to confirm the absence of dementia challenging.

Box 3.7 **Examples of common presentations**

Example One

A 2-year history of progressive change in memory, an ACE score of 70 with poor memory subscores and impaired verbal fluency, together with a scan that shows only temporal atrophy strongly suggests a mild dementia caused by Alzheimer's disease

Example Two

A 5-year history of subtle changes in personality, with lability of mood, emerging lack of empathy, lapses in judgement and relatively well-preserved memory with some semantic loss. An ACE score of 60 with impaired fluency, loss of semantic memory, perseveration noted on tasks throughout, lacking insight into loss of skills strongly suggests a frontotemporal dementia (FTD).

Example Three

An 18-month history of progressive cognitive decline, fluctuant in nature, accompanied by vivid visual hallucinations, and agnosias. A 10-year history of disruption in sleep architecture and rapid eye movement (REM) sleep disturbance, recent changes in gait, and falls. CT head scan shows normal age-related change. ACE score 78, losing points on memory tasks and visuospatial tasks, with preservation of orientation in time and place, fluency and language. Suggests a diagnosis of Lewy body dementia.

Further reading

Hodges J *Cognitive Assessment for Clinicians. Second Edition.* Oxford University Press, 2007.

CHAPTER 4

Early Intervention for Dementia

Bernard Coope and Tanya Jacobs

Worcestershire Health and Care NHS Trust, Worcestershire, UK

> ### OVERVIEW
> - The aim of an Early Intervention Dementia Service is to help those with dementia live well now, and into the future.
> - The focus of this service is helping an individual adapt to the diagnosis and to work with families to build confidence, resilience and skills to face the future.
> - 'Intervention' is the whole process of professional engagement, not just something that happens after a diagnosis.
> - Making a diagnosis is one small part. Sharing it well needs good communication skills and the right setting.
> - Specialists must work with partners who will provide support and advice, and communicate well with primary care.

Introduction

Society's views of dementia are changing and with this the expectations and wishes of our patients are changing too, challenging clinicians and services to adapt. A large proportion of people experiencing the early signs of dementia are now wishing to know if they are developing the condition. Previously, the prevailing view in society was to refrain from discussing dementia – a view shared by most clinicians. A self-perpetuating cycle emerged. Lack of training on dementia for health professionals led to the sense that dementia was not a health care priority, resulting in little recognition of the clinical needs of patients. Two common beliefs have led to the illusion that doing nothing is best.

- People developing dementia are unaware of their impairments and are happy in their ignorance.
- There is nothing that can be done if a diagnosis is made early, as dementia is an incurable condition.

Anyone who has spent time with those developing dementia will know that the first of these is simply untrue. The majority of those with early dementia are only too aware of the changes that are taking place, as are their families. This painful realisation leads to the psychological defense of denial, rather than an organic lack of awareness.

ABC of Dementia, First Edition. Edited by Bernard Coope and Felicity Richards.
© 2014 John Wiley & Sons, Ltd. Published 2014 by John Wiley & Sons, Ltd.

There is now a steady demand from those with early changes in memory and other mental skills for an early assessment and diagnosis. This leads to the second point; what can be done to help those diagnosed early?

Exploring the concept of early intervention in dementia

What is 'early intervention'?

The concept of early intervention started in services for young people, where providing a comprehensive intervention early in development aimed to support a more adaptive future. In mental health, this concept has developed mostly as early intervention for psychosis. Here, supporting an early diagnosis with appropriate treatment, advice and family support can help a person who is developing mental illness maintain the direction of their life, stay in education or employment and maintain important relationships with family and friends. An important part of the concept is that although early intervention may include medical treatment, it is much more than this and consists of using a broad range of psychosocial interventions to help support that person to live well.

The 'Memory Clinic'

As demand for early diagnosis for dementia started to grow, partly driven by the launch of acetylcholinesterase inhibitor therapy, the common service response was the 'Memory Clinic'. There are many different models, all with the same focus – to provide a technically expert diagnosis, sometimes by a multidisciplinary team, then medical treatment if appropriate.

While this model may provide an early diagnosis, patients sometimes report feeling unprepared for the assessment process, with consent sometimes assumed, and a lack of support after the assessment highlighted – after the diagnosis was made, what then? Should the patient be told? Should the relatives be told this confidential information? And in the words of Terry Pratchett, 'After a diagnosis people need to be shown the path, not shown the door'.

Early intervention in dementia

The principal aim of early intervention in dementia is to help those affected by early dementia live as well as possible, both now and into the future. An important consequence of this broad definition is that 'intervention' is not something done to people after the diagnosis. Rather it is the combined impact of contact with services, before, during and after the assessment process.

Another consequence is that 'those affected by early dementia' may include those experiencing the condition and those closest to them. Experience has shown that separating the needs of 'patients' and 'carers' at this point is unhelpful and a distinction that a husband and wife, or mother supported by her children, would not recognise. The Early intervention Service for Dementia in Croydon broke new ground in developing the service model and providing evidence for its effectiveness.

Here, the Early intervention Dementia Service in Worcestershire is described as an example.

The name of the service: mentioning the 'D' word

The Early Intervention Dementia Service in Worcestershire was developed following wide consultation with people with dementia, their families, and partner organisations such as the Alzheimer's Society. An important principle was to help people use the word 'dementia' without being overwhelmed by it. The comparison with the changing use of the word 'cancer' was a frequently quoted example. This view could be summarised in the comment made by one person living with dementia;

How do you expect us to feel comfortable talking about dementia if you can't?

The choice to openly title the service a 'dementia' service came from this, and consequently starts the patient on the long path of adjustment, starting from the point of referral.

The pathway through the Early Intervention Dementia Service is summarised in Box 4.1:

A word on consent

Investigating possible dementia is similar to other areas of medicine. It has the potential to be of great value, but needs to be undertaken either with a patient's consent, or if unable to consent, carried out in that person's best interests – with skill, with proper after care and, above all, with a clear intent to be of help to the patient.

Box 4.1 **The journey through the Early Intervention Dementia Service – The Worcestershire Model**

	Intervention
Before the referral	– Raising public awareness of the service by articles in the press, local radio, posters and fliers. – Liaising with third-sector organisations, e.g. leaving leaflets in Age UK and Alzheimer's Society offices, meeting with Well Check Officers (Age UK) encouraging them to prompt people to visit their GP with concerns about cognition. – Focus on hard-to-reach groups. Awareness raising with referrers including face-to-face meetings and sending out postcard-sized referral criteria cards.
After referral- The Initial Appointment.	– All referrals screened. If accepted, the person is offered an initial appointment at home. Appointment is generally conducted away from a clinical setting, with the focus on promoting choice and control. An individual may feel more empowered to have this appointment in an environment that is familiar and comfortable. The allocated practitioner (normally a nurse) undertakes this visit and remains a constant throughout the person's engagement with the service. – The nature of assessment is discussed and the possibility of a dementia diagnosis is openly explored. It can be useful to talk about the meaning of the term 'dementia', its symptoms and causes at this point, especially if people have preconceived ideas or fears about the condition. It is also an opportunity to point out the possible advantages of an early diagnosis and potential implications. – Choice and consent gathered; to have the assessment, whether to hear the outcome, or consent to share information with others. Experience in Worcestershire is that 97% express the wish to be told the diagnosis in the presence of their family. – For those who choose not to proceed, they are informed verbally about the process for re-referral and a letter is sent reminding them of this and the issues discussed during the initial appointment.
Assessment	– See Chapter 3. Usually in a clinic setting. – Patients and families know what to expect. A history and examination of cognitive skills carried out by a doctor and a nurse. Brain imaging usually arranged. Further detailed neuropsychological assessment, if indicated. Opportunity for families/carers to speak separately if necessary.
Discussion of results	– 'Honest and open' discussion of results, usually with family in accordance with expressed consent of patient. In an outpatient setting, or at home if the patient wishes. Enough detail to clarify the reason and nature of the diagnosis, for example, showing a person their brain imaging. Medication initiated if appropriate. Conversation summarised in personal letter to the patient.
Post diagnostic intervention	– Coordinated and mostly provided by the same nurse who conducted the initial assessment. The aim is to enhance personal adaptation and family resilience.

Intervention	
	– Emotional support for person diagnosed and family. Exploration of the diagnosis both verbally and with written information. Support along with adjusting to the diagnosis can vary and differ considerably between patients and relatives. Consider introduction of Admiral Nurses (Box 4.2) and/or team psychologist for more intense support. – Advice and information, supported by dementia advisor and partners such as Alzheimer's Society. Individualised, especially in non-Alzheimer's disease dementia and younger people. – Support for working age dementia. Addressing social issues including employment or applications for relevant benefits. Addressing the needs of children – liaising with schools and children's services. Providing information about the working age Dementia Café. Links to ongoing sources of peer support, for example, Dementia Café (Box 4.2) and dementia Internet forums. – Carers – referrals to Social Services for a carers' assessment. This can include contingency planning in the event of carer absence and exploration of respite opportunities. Linking carers with voluntary support agencies who can provide further emotional and practical support and access to educational sessions. Making links with dementia support groups. – Identify social needs – referrals to social services for care packages. – Financial, legal and benefit advice – for example, discussion about simplifying finances setting up direct debits. Information about Lasting Power of Attorney (LPA) and how to apply for this. Support with applying for Attendance Allowance – requesting benefits check from Age UK. – Development of skills for continuing to live well, supported by Occupational Therapist and support worker. Functional assessment to establish level of ability and development of strategies to aid daily function and independence e.g. assistive technology. Provided individually or at 'Living well with Dementia' days (see Box 4.2). – Thinking about the future. Encouraging consideration of wishes for the future- via informal discussions or formalised with LPAs and Advance Statements (See Chapter 12) Driving advice. Most people with early dementia still able to drive safely but diagnosis must be communicated to the Driving and Vehicle Licensing Agency DVLA. See Chapter 12. Arrange an in car driving assessment if concerns are identified. Explore alternative modes of transport and support with confidence to access public transport.
Liaising with Primary Care	– Promotion of health lifestyle – identify possible opportunities to improve physical, mental and social activity. Liaising with primary care regarding possible impact of impaired cognition on physical health to coordinate joint management plans, for example, diabetic services, dieticians and pharmacies. – Dental advice. Dental care can be hard to provide in more severe dementia and dental pain can be hard to detect and treat. Good dental health at this point may prevent future problems. – Clear communication regarding diagnosis and intervention with primary care. – Review of effectiveness of acetyl cholinesterase inhibitors after three months.
Discharge from Early Intervention Team	Most people discharged after approximately three months. Personal letter sent to the patient. Letter to GP suggesting follow-up plan and referral route if specialist care is needed in the future.

If the person can give consent, then it is important not only to discuss the process of assessment but also what the possible outcome might be. This also gives an opportunity to find out if the patient wishes to be informed of the assessment's outcome, that is, the possibility of receiving a diagnosis of dementia. If a person lacks the capacity, then assessment must by law be in their best interests and this has to be demonstrated. The assumption must be that a person is capable to give informed consent, unless there is evidence to the contrary.

The Evolving Service Model

If the question is 'What can be done to help this person with dementia and those around live as well as possible?' then there may be more than one answer. The Early Intervention for Dementia model will continue to improve and change. It will need to adapt to growing demand within the context of financial constraint, shaped by the need to be both of high quality and cost-effective. Some likely themes for future debates are listed below.

(i) **Prevention and disease modification**

There is epidemiological and pathological evidence of potentially modifiable risk factors for dementia. These include vascular risk factors, diet, physical activity and depression. Some clinicians are already proposing that interventions targeted at early diagnosis (e.g. cognitive behavioural strategies aimed at preventing future depression) will alter the future course of dementia in a cost-effective way, although there is little current evidence to support this. In a similar way, medications are often reported as being disease modifying, 'staving off the condition for years', rather than correctly outlining the limited efficacy and only modest symptomatic benefit as the evidence suggests. Future technology developments and a growing evidence base will hopefully lead to changes in this area.

(ii) **Primary or Secondary care?**

The process of pre-assessment discussion, consent, assessment and diagnosis sharing is a lengthy one. In the Worcestershire model described earlier, it takes a total of $2\frac{1}{2}$ hours of face-to-face clinical work to get to this point. Then there follows a period of post diagnosis work. This is not a realistic expectation for primary care, but the work could be done within a GP surgery. This can provide a familiar setting to patients and also help joint working with the primary care team. As long as the skills and time are available, the work is not the exclusive domain of any one professional group.

(iii) **To discharge or not discharge?**

The majority of people seen by the Early Intervention Service are in the early stages of their illness path. They benefit from the post-diagnostic support offered and the involvement and signposting to voluntary sector organizations. It is common and more than acceptable to these individuals to be discharged back to their GP. However, a number of people may need to be referred to the Community Mental Health Team if risk is an issue or more comprehensive follow-up is required.

Conclusion

If a person is developing dementia they may benefit from the opportunity to have this clarified in the setting of an intervention that maximises choice and consent and actively engages with families. Making the diagnosis well, sharing it well and then supporting those affected by the diagnosis to live well, now and to the end of their life, are principles that challenge health care professionals to learn new skills and practices that go far beyond diagnostic assessment (Box 4.2).

Box 4.2 **Examples of support following a dementia diagnosis**

Dementia Advisors

Dementia advisors work closely with the service during post-diagnostic intervention and also act as a point of contact following discharge. They offer signposting, advice and information to people experiencing memory loss or who have received a diagnosis of dementia.

Admiral Nurses

Registered mental health nurses specialise in dementia care. Their primary role is to support families and carers of people with dementia. They use a number of interventions to provide practical and emotional support and help people develop skills to enhance well-being and maintain relationships.

Dementia café

Organised by the voluntary sector, for example, Age UK or Alzheimer's Society. A forum for people with dementia and their carers to meet with others and support each other. Relaxed and friendly environment and often attended by guest speakers addressing issues relevant to dementia.

Living well with dementia days

Organised jointly by the Early Intervention Dementia Service and Admiral Nursing Team. Aimed at patients who have recently received a diagnosis of dementia and their families, friends and carers. Designed to be a positive day focusing on living well with dementia. Includes a series of short talks and a chance to meet professionals and organisations who work in the local area.

CHAPTER 5

Drug Treatment

Solmaz Sadaghiani

Worcestershire Health and Care NHS Trust, Worcestershire, UK

> **OVERVIEW**
> - Two classes of treatment are licensed with the aim of improving cognition in dementia.
> - Medications are for symptomatic relief, and have not been shown to have disease-modifying properties.
> - Benefits are often modest, with some patients gaining no perceived benefit from medications.
> - Side effects of cognitive enhancers may limit tolerability.
> - Continued treatment should be guided by evidence of more gain than harm, and by patient choice.

Introduction

Despite continued research into dementia, few treatment options are available for cognitive symptoms. None of them halt or prevent deterioration, and their use is often governed by tolerability and efficacy. Cognitive enhancers, such as acetylcholinesterase inhibitors (AChE inhibitors – donepezil, rivastigmine and glantamine) and memantine are discussed in detail in this chapter.

Ethical considerations

When considering any treatment options, our aim should always be to enable the individual and the carers to live well with the dementia by improving quality of life. Depending on the underlying pathology of the dementia syndrome, treatment with cognitive enhancers such as AChE inhibitors or memantine can be considered.

People who notice a benefit from cognitive enhancers may experience symptomatic relief from cognitive and behavioural symptoms. These can manifest as improvements in motivation, concentration and general alertness but can come at the expense of certain side effects. Indeed, these medications will not be suitable in all cases.

As with all prescribing, a balance needs to be struck between risks and benefits. Where the occurrence of adverse side effects are determined to outweigh the possible benefits, consideration should be given to discontinuation or deciding not to commence the medication at all.

ABC of Dementia, First Edition. Edited by Bernard Coope and Felicity Richards.
© 2014 John Wiley & Sons, Ltd. Published 2014 by John Wiley & Sons, Ltd.

Careful discussion of these issues with the patient and carers is required to manage expectations from the outset, without falsely raising hopes and to dissuade from the notion that cognitive enhancers will halt disease progression.

Available medications

Acetylcholinesterase inhibitors (AChE inhibitors)

The cholinergic hypothesis of Alzheimer's disease (AD) is based on the observation that cognitive deterioration results from progressive loss of cholinergic neurons and decreasing levels of acetylcholine (Ach) in the brain, which these medications help to increase. Three AChE inhibitors are currently licensed in the UK for the treatment of dementia in AD:

Donepezil
Rivastigmine
Galantamine

In addition, rivastigmine is licensed in the treatment of mild-to-moderate dementia in Parkinson's disease. AChE inhibitors differ in pharmacological action (Box 5.1).

Memantine

Memantine is a voltage-dependent, moderate-affinity, uncompetitive N-methyl-D-aspartate (NMDA) receptor antagonist that blocks the effects of pathologically elevated tonic levels of glutamate, which may lead to neuronal dysfunction (Box 5.1).

Efficacy

AChE inhibitors and memantine can offer symptomatic treatment and there is no evidence to suggest that survival is affected. Treatment with AChE inhibitors can produce modest improvements in cognition, functional and behavioural symptoms as well as lowering care giver burden and delaying institutionalisation.

Absence of 'close comparison' studies suggests that available medications should be assumed to have parallel efficacy against cognitive symptoms. Each of the AChE inhibitors offers benefits over best supportive care.

Under clinical trial conditions if AChE inhibitors are given at optimal doses, roughly one-third of people would be expected to

Box 5.1 **Characteristics of cognitive enhancers**

Cognitive enhancer	Mechanism of action	Dosing	Formulation	Adverse effects
Donepezil	Selectively inhibits AChE	Once daily	Tablets Orodispersible tablets	Nausea Vomiting Dizziness Insomnia, diarrhoea Urinary incontinence Muscle cramps Fatigue Syncope Hallucinations
Rivastigmine	Affects both AChE + BuChE	Twice daily (oral) Once daily (patch) Prolonged titration schedules	Capsules Oral solution Transdermal patch	As given
Galantamine	Selectively inhibits AChE Acts as anallosteric ligand at nicotinic Ach receptors	Once-daily controlled release formulation Twice daily Prolonged titration schedules	Capsules Tablets Oral solution	As given
Memantine	NMDA (N-methyl-D-aspartate) receptor partial antagonist	5 mg od and then increased in steps of 5 mg at weekly intervals to a maximum of 20 mg daily	Tablets Oral drops	Agitation Falls, dizziness Accidental injury influenza-like symptoms Headache Diarrhoea Constipation Somnolence Hypertension

cardiac conduction disturbance, such as sinoatrial or atrioventricular block.

The advice by all three manufacturers has therefore been that the drugs should be used with caution in patients with cardiovascular disease or in those taking a combination of an AChE inhibitor and bradycardic drugs, for example, digoxin and beta blockers. Care should also be taken in those with symptoms of postural hypotension or syncope. Given that the incidence of cardiovascular side effects is deemed to be low, the value of routine electrocardiogram (ECG) is debatable and they are not routinely recommended by National Institute of Clinical Excellence (NICE).

Peptic ulcer disease and gastrointestinal (GI) bleeding secondary to increased gastric acid secretion due to increased cholinergic activity may be a possibility especially in predisposed individuals.

Donepezil and galantamine are metabolised by cytochrome 2D6 and 3A4, so drug levels may be altered by other drugs affecting the function of these enzymes.

Dosing

When treating those with a poor memory, it is best to keep dosing schedules simple. Once-daily treatment is best. Wherever possible, carers should be aware of the treatment being started and asked if they can help support compliance.

Cognitive enhancers and behavioural and psychological symptoms of dementia

Trial of AChE inhibitors is an appropriate pharmacological strategy as part of a wider care plan for behavioural and psychological symptoms of dementia, as discussed in Chapter 8. Effects seem apparent only after several weeks of treatment. However, AChE inhibitors can also lead to an increase in agitation and aggressive behaviours, so caution should be exercised. In dementia with Lewy bodies, AChE inhibitors may help with visual hallucinations.

Of note, depression is common in dementia, considered both as a cause and a consequence. The prevalence of comorbid depression is estimated to be 30–50%. Symptoms can occur at all stages of illness. A biopsychosocial approach should be used, with medication playing its part.

Vascular dementia

In vascular dementia, the underlying pathology is ischaemic damage to the brain, causing cognitive impairment and behavioural disturbance. The management remedies are currently limited and the initial strategy is to establish causative factors and optimise underlying risk factors for cerebrovascular disease.

Daily aspirin may delay the course of the disease. The management of vascular risk factors may include a change of diet, stopping smoking, managing hypertension, optimising diabetic control and increasing exercise.

None of the currently available medication is formally licensed in the UK for vascular dementia as there is insufficient evidence to support widespread use of these agents.

improve and around one-third would be expected not to deteriorate. These estimations appear to be echoed in practice. Memantine can have a small beneficial effect at 6 months in moderate-to-severe AD. Statistically significant effects were detected on cognition, activities of daily living and behaviour.

Current treatment guidance in the UK is for monotherapy.

Adverse effects and interaction

Excess cholinergic stimulation can lead to nausea, vomiting, dizziness, insomnia and diarrhoea (Box 5.1).

Vagotonic effects can lead to bradycardia. This may be of importance in patients with sick sinus syndrome or other supraventricular

In clinical practice, the situation may be less clear. A mixture of Alzheimer's disease and vascular disease is very common, so the presence of vascular disease does not mean the absence of Alzheimer's disease. When faced with a patient with a clinical dementia and vascular disease on a scan, mixed dementia is likely and a pragmatic approach may be to try cholinesterase inhibitors and assess for benefit.

Guidance from the National Institute of Clinical Excellence (NICE)

In the UK, the use of AChE inhibitors and memantine is covered by specific NICE Guidance TA217 published in March 2011.

The three AChE inhibitors, donepezil, galantamine and rivastigmine, are recommended as options for managing mild-to-moderate Alzheimer's disease.

Memantine is recommended as an option for managing people with moderate Alzheimer's disease who are intolerant of or have a contraindication to AChE inhibitors, or who have severe Alzheimer's disease.

Only specialists in the care of patients with dementia (i.e. psychiatrists including those specialising in learning disability, neurologists, and physicians specialising in the care of older people) should initiate treatment. Carers' views on the patient's condition at baseline should be sought.

Treatment should be continued only when it is considered to be having a worthwhile effect on cognitive, global, functional or behavioural symptoms.

Patients who continue on treatment should be reviewed regularly using cognitive, global, functional and behavioural assessment. Treatment should be reviewed by an appropriate specialist team, unless there are locally agreed protocols for shared care. Carers' views on the patient's condition at follow-up should be sought.

If prescribing an AChE inhibitor (donepezil, galantamine or rivastigmine), treatment should normally be started with the drug with the lowest acquisition cost.

Criticisms of the guidance

At the time of publication, there was considerable controversy about the restricted use of the medications. There are two main criticisms:

1 **Cost-effectiveness**. At the time of publication of the NICE guidance, the cost of AChE inhibitors was high, approximately £60 for a four-week supply of 5 mg donepezil, for example. The stipulation that only specialists should initiate treatment was intended to avoid unnecessary cost to the NHS of inappropriate prescribing. Now that generic formulations are available, cost has reduced substantially, approximately £2 per month for 5 mg donepezil.
2 **Evidence of use in severe dementia**. Since the publication, more evidence has been put forth that indicates a benefit from AChE inhibitors in severe dementia.

These two changes put together raise serious questions about the need for regular follow-up and measurement of cognition, a process that uses far more NHS resource in the form of clinician time than it could possibly save. With evidence of effectiveness across the whole spectrum of severity of Alzheimer's disease, there is no longer ground to stop treatment unless by patient choice or due to adverse effects. Therefore, repeatedly measuring cognition with the intent of stopping cholinesterase inhibitors when dementia becomes severe can no longer be supported. Patients can thus avoid the indignity of repeated testing and specialists can use their time to see those with more pressing need.

Thinking about treatment – what should be discussed with the patient and carer?

Despite potential difficulties in communication between clinician and patient, the process of gaining informed consent when reaching a decision remains of paramount importance. In some cases where capacity is an issue, consent will ideally need to be sought from the carer and a number of areas should be covered. These include the following:

- The chance of benefit
- The chance of side effects
- The symptomatic rather than disease-modifying nature of treatment.

Box 5.2 Drugs to avoid

Drugs	Example	Comment
Analgesics	Narcotic	Sedation
Antiarrhythmics	Disopyramide	Negative inotrope anticholinergic
Antidepressants	Tricyclics (TCAs)	Orthostatic hypotension→falls
		Anticholinergic Increase confusion
Antiemetics	Promethazine	Cause EPSE (Extra pyramidal side effects)
Antiparkinsonian	Procyclidine, Benztropine Levodopa	Anticholinergic Exacerbating psychotic symptoms
Antipsychotics	See preceding text	See preceding text
Anxiolytics	Benzodiazepines	If for anxiety, consider short-acting Lorazepam
Gastrointestinal/ urinary antispasmodics	Atropine, Oxybutynin, Tolterodine	Anticholinergic
Antihistamines	Promethazine	Anticholinergic Sedation

Drugs to avoid in cognitive decline

Older people with dementia are more prone to developing drug-induced cognitive impairment. Medications with strong anticholinergic (AC) side effects are well known for this. In order to achieve maximum therapeutic effect with AChE inhibitors, combinations with anticholinergic agents should be avoided as these are known to have an opposing mechanism of action (Box 5.2). General practioners can help by reviewing polypharmacy and by remaining vigilant for some of the more commonly prescribed drugs that are known to be inappropriate, for example; amitriptyline for insomnia, betahistidine for vertigo and oxybutynin for urinary frequency.

Conclusion

Medication options for dementia are limited. AChE inhibitors and memantine may provide some symptomatic relief (both cognitively and non-cognitively); however, they are commonly associated with intolerability and lack of efficacy. Discussions surrounding their use should take place with the person with dementia and family/carers, and decisions should be made in an informed way. These medications may play a small part in helping a person live well with their dementia.

Further reading

Boehringer SK, Cupp M. *Drugs to Avoid in Patients with Dementia. Pharmacist's Letter and Prescriber's Letter.* 2008;Vol. **24**:Number 240510 http://www.albany.edu/sph/coned/sta/attachment_13_medications.pdf

Drug information online. *Donepezil Official FDA Information, Side Effects and Uses.* 2013. http://www.drugs.com/pro/donepezil.html

Howard R, McShane R, lindesay J, et al. Donepezil and memantine for moderate-to-severe Alzheimer's disease. *N Engl J Med* 2012; **366**:893–903

National institute of Clinical Excellence. *Donepezil, Glantamine, Rivastigmine and Memantine for the Treatment of Alzheimer's Disease. Review of NICE Technology Appraisal Guidance 111.* NICE, London, 2011. http://www.nice.org.uk/nicemedia/live/13419/53619/53619.pdf

Taylor D, Paton C, Kapur S. *The Maudsley. Prescribing Guidelines in Psychiatry. Eleventh Edition.* Wiley-Blackwell, London, 2012.

CHAPTER 6

Dementia and Families

Jenny La Fontaine

Association for Dementia Studies, University of Worcester, Henwick Grove, Worcestershire, UK

OVERVIEW

- Family relationships are of considerable importance to people with dementia.
- A range of complex factors influence the family experience of dementia including previous and current relationship quality.
- Both satisfaction and challenges are evident in family caregiving, but risk factors influencing negative outcomes are frequently unique to each person involved in caregiving.
- A tailored assessment to identify the needs of family caregivers is a necessary aspect of effective practice in dementia care.
- Families benefit from psychosocial interventions, in particular multicomponent interventions that include psychological support, information and education.

Introduction

Family life forms an everyday part of our existence; families can provide important opportunities to meet our needs for intimacy, love and affection, belongingness, challenge, security and celebration. Families can also provide a source of strength in times of need, providing practical, emotional, financial and spiritual assistance.

Box 6.1 **Exercise 1**

Consider your answers to the following questions:

- Write down the people who you consider to be in your family
- Spend a few minutes writing down the things that you are going to be doing in your personal life over the next few weeks or months.

In answering the first question, it is likely that the people you have identified as family will be defined as such by virtue of their blood relationship to you; others may be considered by you to be 'family' because of the bond you experience with them and are relationships

such as marriage, civil partnerships or friendships. Who we define as family has significant variability from person to person, and represents the heterogeneity of family life in the 21st century.

In considering your answer to the second question, it is likely that a number of the activities or events that you have identified will involve the people you consider to be family, which underlines the significant roles that family has in our everyday lives, through the life course. This is no less true for older people, with research identifying that family relationships are of greater significance, influencing feelings of being well, psychologically, spiritually, physically and emotionally.

Dementia and families

Two-thirds of people who live with dementia in the UK live at home, frequently with family members, who either live with them or nearby. Families are recognised to be the primary source of support for people living with dementia, and are fundamental to enabling them to remain at home. Even when a person with dementia is admitted to a care home setting, the family continues to be important in their lives, promoting well-being, enabling the person to maintain links with the family and community and in supporting staff to care for them.

Dementia impacts upon intimate relationships, including those in long-term partnerships or marriage. Furthermore, the involvement of family is not limited to spousal relationships, with research evidence highlighting that a range of family relationships are affected, including adult children and grandchildren.

As with other chronic and life-limiting illnesses, it is necessary to acknowledge that dementia impacts upon the whole family. Accordingly, there is a need to develop and deliver effective interventions that can enable families to adapt to and prevent negative outcomes such as depression. In order to achieve this, it is necessary to understand the family experience of dementia, and to consider in what ways services can respond to the needs of families affected by dementia.

The family experience of dementia

Ros and Roy Dibble describe their personal experience of managing the impact of dementia upon their lives. Ros who is 59,

---

ABC of Dementia, First Edition. Edited by Bernard Coope and Felicity Richards.
© 2014 John Wiley & Sons, Ltd. Published 2014 by John Wiley & Sons, Ltd.

has a diagnosis of posterior cortical atrophy (PCA), a variant of Alzheimer's disease.

From Roy Dibble, Ros's husband: 'We have been struggling to start a new way of living/working since Ros was diagnosed as having PCA over a year ago. PCA leaves the person with difficulties of spatial awareness as well as memory problems and Ros has difficulties when driving (she has given up), writing, using the keyboard, walking down steps or stairs or dressing.

Our journey through the process of coping and managing the onset of dementia might be compared with the way in which most of us were taught history at school. We had a Before Crisis (BC) when there was a period of concern that there might be something wrong with Ros, then a realisation that this was a real problem followed by recognition that something would have to be done and that the doctor (GP) would have to be consulted. Looking back, the BC period was as long as three years as we struggled to come to terms with the problem plus the natural reluctance to seek help and visit the doctor.

This was followed by the After Diagnosis (AD) period, which has now lasted for well over a year. Despite the help we have received, Ros has had a constant battle trying to come to terms with a massive loss of independence, largely as a result of not being able to drive a car and the frustration of not being able to perform the simplest tasks that were carried out with ease only a few months before. Having to rely on others has been particularly difficult for a lively, outgoing individual such as Ros.'

For Roy as the carer/partner, there has been an equal loss of freedom and independence coupled with a need to take on, and in some cases to learn, to do many things that were previously managed by Ros.

'We have tried to ensure that we do as much as possible together in the form of joint tasks in order to keep things as normal as possible. It is inevitable that the situation looks bleak from time to time and that there are good days and bad days. Perhaps the most difficult issue to cope with is the knowledge that the medication only slows down the process of deterioration which results in the constant self-questioning of "why did it happen to me?," "what will happen in the future?" and "how long will it take?" We have learnt that it is vital that the carer keeps calm and encourages the partner to keep cheerful and to continue to do all of the things that they are able to do as stopping often leads to an inability to continue to carry out the task.

Our constant plea to each other during the AD period is to try to continue to carry on with as much of our former life as possible doing as many of the things that we feel able to do. Maintaining a sense of humour and laughing at adversity is vital. It is rarely possible to do new things or to go beyond what we define as our "comfort zone" but it is essential that we keep trying but not pushing to achieve impossible objectives.'

For Ros, listening to music, walking to the village shop alone to buy small items, going to the post office or supermarket, or helping Roy prepare the dinner are essential means of retaining her capabilities. She has also contributed to work on Alzheimer's and dementia in a number of areas and finds that talking to people directly or by telephone both helpful and therapeutic. Tiredness, stress and anxiety are the key dangers to be avoided at all costs as far as Ros is concerned.

'Every day brings new challenges that have to be managed as best they can. The illness has introduced many difficulties for both of us but we have both made adjustments to our previous highly active lives in order to cope with the new situation.'

Box 6.2 Exercise 2

Ros's and Roy's description highlights a number of key issues for them in managing the impact of dementia upon their lives; you might wish to list these for yourself, before reading further.

Ros's and Roy's experience highlights that recognising something is wrong is often a long and slow process. Many families describe this as a traumatic time, in which relationships can become strained as people experience difficulties in understanding what is happening. Reasons for delaying help seeking include stigma and the belief that the cause is normal ageing. This is likely to be more prolonged when family members have differing perspectives or difficulty acknowledging that something might be wrong.

Having received a diagnosis, the quality of the previous and current relationship, and the way in which the impact is negotiated by all parties in the relationship will affect how the illness is coped with. Ros and Roy are able to talk together and discuss their situation, including considering potentially painful questions about the future. This is not the case for all families, particularly where the previous relationship has been poor, and where open communication has not been a feature of the relationship.

The strategies used by family members are likely to include maintaining valued aspects of relationships, including shared activities and also time apart in independent activities. For couples, this may also include maintaining intimacy, including sexual intimacy. However, such strategies may become less possible, particularly as dementia progresses, and the person with dementia is less able to actively engage with such processes. In this context, family members may find themselves acting independently of the person with dementia in their efforts to manage the impact, and finding the challenges of this particularly complex and potentially distressing.

Even in the early experience of dementia, considerable adaptation is necessary. This includes changes in roles and independence in everyday lives. Such changes are likely to challenge even the strongest of relationships, and while many family members involved in caregiving identify satisfaction in their role, it is nevertheless recognised that for many, negative outcomes also occur. These include depression, chronic and acute stress, poor physical health including heart disease, and admission to long-term care of the person with dementia. Such outcomes arise from a complex interplay of a number of factors, as identified in Table 6.1.

Assessment of families and family members in caregiving relationships

The above highlights the need for health care professionals to take seriously the well-being and needs of family members as well as the person with dementia. A failure to acknowledge and respond to the well-being needs of all family members increases the likelihood

Table 6.1 Factors contributing to or mediating the risk of negative outcomes.

Psychological factors	Physical factors	Relational factors
Resilience	Sleeplessness	Quality of previous and current relationship
Service use	Self-care	Communication styles
The meaning of changes in behaviour	Chronic and multiple acute stressors	Quality of social support networks
The well-being of the person with dementia	Depression is linked to cardiovascular pathology	The meanings and motivations behind caring
The caregiving context	Psychological factors combine to increase risk of poor physical health	The experience of family and community values and beliefs
The severity of the dementia		The quality of family support
The ability to develop strategies and find solutions		
The type of dementia		

Data from Elvish R, Lever S-J, Johnstone J, et al. *Psychological Interventions for Carers of People with Dementia: A Systematic Review of Quantitative and Qualitative Evidence*. British Association for Counselling and Psychotherapy. 2012 http://www.bacp.co.uk/research/Systematic_Reviews_and_Publications/dementia_carers.php

of an early admission to a care home setting for the person with dementia. This support begins with providing an assessment for family members involved in caregiving.

The factors influencing negative outcomes are unique to each family caregiver. Therefore, assessments need to be planned carefully, with interventions targeted at the risk factors and outcomes related to that caregiver. While there may be specific groups of family caregivers that are at greater risk of poor outcomes, for example, caregiving for people with younger onset dementia, or for partners, it is necessary to recognise the high level of individual variability in the family experience of caregiving. A multidimensional approach to assessment should be taken. This may begin with a brief assessment identifying areas of concern, which can prompt a referral to appropriate agencies who can deliver a detailed and tailored assessment.

Interventions with families affected by dementia

Interventions that are most effective for family members living with dementia are multicomponent and tailored to the individual needs of the family caregiver; involve them in deciding what forms of intervention are required; involve the person with dementia in order to address well-being needs and provide opportunities to address the relational context in which caregiving takes place.

Multicomponent interventions include

- a combination of individual, family and group interventions depending on the needs and wishes of the family caregiver and the person with dementia, and
- are designed to address the development of coping strategies and enhance resilience, which include the family caregiver as an active participant in this process, and
- cover the delivery of a range of possible processes, including
  - providing emotional support and assistance
  - enhancing family and support networks
  - developing communication skills and strategies
  - self-care strategies
  - knowledge concerning support services
  - knowledge of dementia and strategies to understand and cope with distressed behaviour of the person with dementia
  - meaningful activity and occupation
  - stress management techniques.

Conclusion

Family relationships commonly assist us to maintain well-being, manage life's challenges and support in times of crisis throughout our lives. Family relationships are of considerable importance to people with dementia, because without them the opportunities to experience well-being, and furthermore to remain at home, are significantly reduced. The experience of dementia for families involves a complex interplay between the impact of dementia; the previous and current relationship quality; the strategies that are used to manage the impact of the changes, and the meaning of the changes for all involved, including the person with dementia.

Both satisfaction and challenges are evident in family caregiving, but risk factors influencing negative outcomes are frequently unique to each person involved in caregiving, and require a tailored assessment in which the family member's needs are assessed and their perspective sought on what might be helpful. Families benefit from psychosocial interventions, which include tailored psychological and emotional support as well as information and education.

It is imperative that practitioners recognise that working with families is a fundamental part of work with people who live with dementia. Failing to address the needs of family members has significant and deleterious outcomes for all family members, including increased levels of physical and mental health difficulties and the likelihood that a person with dementia will be placed in long-term care.

Acknowledgement

The author expresses her gratitude to Ros and Roy Dibble for their contribution.

Further reading

Balducci C, Mnich E, McKee KJ, et al. Negative impact and positive value in caregiving: validation of the COPE index in a 6-country sample of carers. *Gerontologist* 2008; **48**:276–286.

Elvish R, Lever S-J, Johnstone J, Cawley R, Keady J. *Psychological Interventions for Carers of People with Dementia: A Systematic Review of Quantitative and Qualitative Evidence*. British Association for Counselling and Psychotherapy, 2012.

Keady J Nolan M. The dynamics of dementia: working together, working separately or working alone? In: Nolan M, Lundh U, Grant G, and Keady J (eds), *Partnerships in Family Care: Understanding the Caregiving Career*. Open University Press: Buckingham, 2003: 15–32.

Rolland J. *Families, Illness and Disability, An Integrative Treatment Model*. Basic Books: New York, 1994.

Zarit S. *Assessment of Family Caregivers: A Research Perspective, Family Care Giver Alliance, Care Giver Assessment: Voices and Views from the Field*. 2006; Vol. **2** http://www.caregiver.org/caregiver/jsp/content/pdfs/v2_consensus.pdf (accessed October 2010).

CHAPTER 7

Person-Centred Care

Dawn Brooker

Association for Dementia Studies, University of Worcester, Worcester, UK

OVERVIEW

- There is a risk that people living with dementia who are losing their cognitive powers get treated as if they are 'non-persons'.

- The maintenance of personhood underpins the practice of person-centred care (PCC). The term malignant social psychology describes those episodes where personhood is undermined.

- Good communication skills that support the person with dementia while not undermining their remaining abilities can do much to maintain personhood.

- The VIPS framework for PCC provides a set of reflection points for health care professionals to assess their own practice and to assess the whole organisation approach to the provision of person-centred practice.

- The use of language that de-humanises or stigmatises is to be avoided.

Personhood in dementia

The progressive cognitive impairments that are the hallmark of dementia sometimes make it appear to others that the person is disappearing as the disease progresses. Since the seminal theoretical work of Kitwood in the 1990s, a person-centred approach for understanding the experience of dementia is advocated and has been demonstrated to have a positive impact on well-being. PCC rests on a value base that recognises the personhood of all persons regardless of age or cognitive ability. This challenges the assumption that dementia is the death that leaves the body behind. It requires that those living with dementia are treated as individuals, recognising that all people have a unique history and personality. It also requires that the perspective of the individual is seen as the starting point for care and that empathy with this perspective has its own therapeutic potential. People living with dementia need an enriched social environment that compensates for their impairment and fosters opportunities for ensuring that they have chances for closeness to others. People with dementia have a continuing capacity to experience relative well-being and ill-being, and this is

strongly influenced by the behaviour of others towards them – the psychosocial milieu (Figure 7.1).

Although cognition fails, there are numerous accounts of the person's need for warm human contact if a state of well-being is to be achieved. With the onset of dementia, individuals are very vulnerable to their psychological defences being broken down. As the sense of self breaks down, it becomes increasingly important that it is reinforced by others through the relationships the person with dementia experiences (Figure 7.2).

Malignant Social Psychology

Kitwood described personhood as being undermined when individual needs and rights are not considered, when powerful negative emotions are ignored or invalidated and when increasing isolation from human relationships occurs. He used the phrase Malignant Social Psychology (MSP) as an umbrella term for such episodes, using terms such as intimidation, outpacing, infantilisation, labelling, disparagement, blaming, manipulating, invalidating, disempowering, overpowering, disrupting, objectifying, stigmatising, ignoring, banishing and mocking to illustrate the many ways that personhood can be undermined in non-person-centred care environments. MSP is rarely done with malicious intent. It can become interwoven into the care culture within some organisations and can easily take hold unless constant effort is made to keep it at bay. New staff learn from existing staff how to communicate with people with dementia. If the staff communication style is one that is characterised by the infantilisation and outpacing of people with dementia, then the new staff member is likely to follow this lead. The malignancy in MSP is that it eats away at the personhood of those being cared for and it also spreads very quickly from one member of staff to another. High levels of challenging behaviour, distress or apathy occur more commonly in care situations that are not supportive of personhood.

Positive person work

Personhood can be supported by positive interactions such as those that feature recognition of the person, negotiation, collaboration, a sense of fun, creativity, engagement through the senses, celebration, relaxation, validation, holding, facilitating and enabling the person to be engaged in life. We know that skilled person-centred care

---

ABC of Dementia, First Edition. Edited by Bernard Coope and Felicity Richards.
© 2014 John Wiley & Sons, Ltd. Published 2014 by John Wiley & Sons, Ltd.

"The person with Dementia or the Person with dementia?"

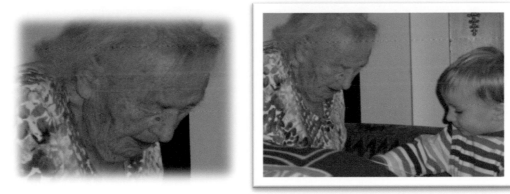

Figure 7.1 Who do you see when you are asked to assess a patient with dementia?

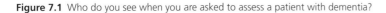

"How you relate to us has a big impact on the course of the disease. You can restore our personhood, and give us a sense of being needed and valued. There is a Zulu saying that is very true. **"A person is a person through others"**. *Give us reassurance, hugs, support, a meaning in life. Value us for what we can still do and be, and make sure we retain social networks. It is very hard for us to be who we once were, so let us be who we are now and realise the effort we are making to function."* Christine Bryden, 2005

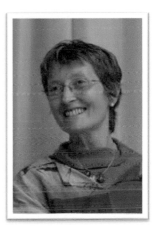

Figure 7.2 One of the richest accounts of what it is like to live with dementia comes from the Australian writer Christine Bryden who was diagnosed with dementia at the age of 46.

and support early on in dementia (such as individualised family assessment, skills training, information, counselling and support) delays care-home admission and improves caregiver mood. We know that skilled person-centred care and support minimises the escalation of problems into behavioural and psychological symptoms of dementia (BPSD). In care homes, we know that people with dementia have better mood and quality of life if they are cared for by staff who communicate well and that staff who are trained in person-centred care decrease agitation levels in high-dependency care-home residents. Sensitive engagement in interaction and personalised activities decreases levels of agitation and ill-being.

Communicating well with people living with dementia

Most of the interventions we make with people with dementia and their families do not rely on the prescription of medication. They rely on good communication. People with dementia face particular challenges in having their voice heard. The cognitive impairment associated with dementia often affects memory function, the ability to use and understand spoken and written language, the ability to

carry out practical everyday tasks, the ability to perceive the world as others do or the ability to plan a course of action. Although there is a decline in cognitive abilities, there is no decline in depth of feeling or the range of emotions that people with dementia experience. Indeed, in many situations, emotions appear stronger than ever. Anger, joy, grief and excitement are often easily accessed. Being aware of the pattern of cognitive deficits and the strength of emotions is a key ingredient in PCC because it enables health care professionals to use communication skills to respond appropriately to individual patients. The aim is to find a response that supports the person with dementia while not undermining their remaining abilities.

Health care professionals can do a great deal to provide the structure that people with dementia need in order to communicate, even when time is limited. The approach to communication will depend on the level and type of cognitive impairment. Some people – particularly early on in their dementia – may have very little problem communicating. It may be enough that the health professional is mindful of summarising regularly, checking out understanding and providing assistance to keep people on track. Other people with much more advanced dementia may have virtually no language at all. In these situations, the person will need a lot more help to ensure their 'voice' gets heard. Many people will fall between these two extremes and the ability to communicate is often sensitive to factors other than the dementia. Factors such as tiredness, lack of hydration and acute illness will have a much bigger impact on communication skills in a person struggling with cognitive impairment. Noisy environments and poor lighting will further exacerbate difficulties. Also, if English is a second language, this often deteriorates more quickly than the mother tongue; therefore, communicating in the correct language is important.

As verbal communication becomes more difficult, attending carefully to the non-verbal behaviour or piecing together fragmented speech becomes increasingly important.

Striking up a good rapport is often not dependent on verbal skills. As verbal abilities are lost, the importance of respectful, warm, accepting human contact through non-verbal channels becomes even more important. Courtesy, respect, friendliness and kindness are usually communicated by non-verbal actions and tone of voice. Also, people with dementia may be more aware of any mismatch between what is being communicated verbally and non-verbally, because of their stronger reliance on non-verbal communication. For example, if the health professional looks annoyed or off-hand in body language or facial expressions, this is what a person with dementia will notice, even if the words are saying something very different (Figure 7.3).

The challenge of providing person-centred care

The concepts in PCC are not easy to articulate and can feel difficult to translate into everyday practice. The VIPS definition of person-centred dementia care attempts to synthesise the different threads of PCC whilst maintaining the sophistication of Kitwood's original theories. This can be summarised in the equation PCC = V + I + P + S. This equation does not give a pre-eminence of any element over another, just that they are all contributory. It also reminds us that we are providing care for very important persons (Figure 7.4).

The VIPS definition was used in the NICE/SCIE guidelines on dementia (Figure 7.5).

The VIPS elements can be used as general guiding principles for health care practitioners to reflect on their interactions with people with dementia and their families. Reflective questions include the following:

- Does my behaviour and the manner in which I am communicating with this person show that I respect, **value** and honour them?
- Am I treating this person as a unique **individual**?
- Am I making a serious attempt to see my actions from the **perspective** of the person I am trying to help? How might my actions be interpreted by this person?
- Does my behaviour and interactions help this person to feel **socially** confident and that they are not alone?

These principles apply in every situation when health care professionals communicate. They apply when giving someone an injection, helping a person use the toilet, assisting a person to complete an advanced care plan or in running a reminiscence group. It is not the task that is person-centred but the way in which that task is done that can make it person-centred or not.

The whole organisation approach

Providing care in a humanistic and person-centred way that really aims to value people living with dementia is a challenge, particularly in care homes and hospitals where frontline care staff themselves may not feel their own personhood is valued. High-level staff turnover, staff shortages and poorly trained staff lead to negative

1. Are patients & families included and involved in conversations or are they talked over and disregarded?

2. Are patients and families shown great respect, courtesy and politeness at all times or are there episodes of telling offs, admonishments and labelling people as difficult?

3. Are patients and families treated with a warm, caring and encouraging attitude or are they treated with indifference and coldness?

4. Do patients and families know that staff take their fears seriously or are people left alone for long periods in emotional distress?

5. Are patients helped with activities such as eating and drinking and personal care when they need it or are they simply done to – often called feeding and toileting?

Figure 7.3 Is the communication style indicative of Malignant Social Psychology or Positive Person Work? Think about your own practice and the services with which you work.

The VIPS definition of person-centred care encompasses:

V A **value** base that asserts the absolute value of all human lives

I An **individualised** approach, recognising uniqueness

P Understanding the world from the **perspective** of the person living with dementia

S Promotion of a positive **social psychology** in which the person living with dementia can experience relative well-being

Figure 7.4 The VIPS definition of person centred care (Brooker, 2007).

The principles of person-centred care underpin good practice in the field of dementia care and they are reflected in many of the recommendations made in the guideline. The principles assert

- The human value of people with dementia, regardless of age or cognitive impairment, and those who care for them
- the individuality of people with dementia, with their unique personality and life experiences among the influences on their response to the dementia
- the importance of the perspective of the person with dementia
- the importance of relationships and interactions with others to the person with dementia, and their potential for promoting well-being.

Figure 7.5 NICE clinical guidelines on Dementia: Supporting people with dementia and their carers in health and social care.

VALUING; The directors, senior team
V1 the vision is clear on dementia
V2 human resource management
V3 management ethos
V4 training & staff development
V5 the service environments
V6 quality assurance, improvement & governance

INDIVIDUALISED; clinical leads
I1 care pathways and planning
I2 regular reviews
I3 personal possessions
I4 individual preferences
I5 life story work
I6 activity & occupation

PERSPECTIVE; shift leaders
P1 skilled communication
P2 empathy , risk & decisions
P3 physical environment managed
P4 physical health needs
P5 challenging behaviour, BPSD
P6 advocacy

SOCIAL RELATIONSHIP; everyone
S1 inclusion
S2 respect
S3 warmth
S4 validation
S5 enabling
S6 family & community

Figure 7.6 The VIPS framework for implementing person centred care across a whole organization. Leadership at different levels is required to ensure the building blocks and structures are in place to support the delivery of personn-centred care at an individual level.

quality of life for care-home residents. Staff who feel demoralised, burnt out and stressed are unlikely to be able to take the care to communicate in the respectful, warm and inclusive way that is required in person-centred care. To achieve person-centred care as part of regular care in care homes and hospitals demands the involvement of staff at all levels of the organisation. The VIPS framework provides a checklist of 24 indicators that care providers can use as a benchmark to assess the person-centredness of their service. This provides concrete examples of the practice that should be in place within any care organisation that claims to provide person-centred dementia care (Figure 7.6).

Person-centred care requires sign-up to working in this way across the whole care provider organisation if it is to be sustained over any length of time. Particular elements require leadership at different levels. Valuing requires leadership from those responsible for leading the organisation at a senior level. Individual care requires leadership, particularly from those responsible for setting care standards and procedures within the organisation. Perspectives and social environment require leadership for those responsible for the day-to-day management and provision of care. This is also available as a free website (www.carefitforvips.co.uk), which enables care-home providers to assess how well they are delivering care against the 24 indicators and helps them identify priorities for improvement. It also contains extensive information and resources covering all aspects of person-centred dementia care alongside online quality improvement cycles to plan, test and record ideas for improvements.

Finally, a word about labels

Health care professionals sometimes have a habit of using labels to describe people.

Although not intentional, this can promote the sort of malignant social psychology that Kitwood wrote about all those years ago as undermining personhood. Referring to people as bed blockers, wanderers, shouters or dements undermines the humanity of people who are using health care. Even terms such as the elderly (rather than older people) or dementia sufferers (rather than people living with dementia) promote a certain image that most people would prefer not to be associated with. The language that is used by health care professionals has a powerful impact on those living with dementia, their families and other staff involved in care.

> "Please don't call us 'dementing' – we are still people separate from our disease, we just have a disease of the brain. If I had cancer you would not refer to me as 'cancerous' would you?" Christine Bryden, 2005.

Further reading

Brooker, D. *Person-Centred Dementia Care: Making Services Better*. Jessica Kingsley, London, 2007.

Bryden, C. *Dancing with Dementia: My Story of Living Positively with Dementia*. Jessica Kingsley, London, 2005.

Greenblat, C. *Love, Loss and Laughter: Seeing Alzheimer's Differently*. Lyons Press, Guildford, CT, 2012.

Kitwood, T. *Dementia Reconsidered: The Person Comes First*. Buckingham, Open University Press, 1997.

Worcestershire Health and Care NHS Trust. *Stand by Me: DVD Assisted Education Resource for Promoting Good Communication with People Living with Dementia and their Families*. Association for Dementia Studies, University of Worcester, Worcester, 2011.

Useful websites

Care fit for VIPS: www.carefitforvips.co.uk

Social Care Institute for Excellence: Dementia Gateway www.scie.org.uk/publications/dementia

CHAPTER 8

Behavioural and Psychological Symptoms of Dementia (BPSD)

Dhanjeev Marrie and Sally Williams

Worcestershire Health and Care NHS Trust, Worcestershire, UK

OVERVIEW

- Challenging behaviours in dementia are a major health and social care issue.
- Behavioural change and psychological symptoms of dementia (BPSD) experienced by people with dementia are a considerable source of caregiver distress and are strongly associated with care home placement.
- Comprehensive assessment is required along with close collaboration with carers and key professionals.
- Management of challenging behaviours can be varied and range from watchful waiting to targeted interventions for specific symptoms.

Introduction

In order to understand an individual's behaviours, we need to understand the individual. Human behaviour or understandable psychological distress itself is not an illness, but if a change occurs in someone's behaviour or mental state with a diagnosis of dementia, 'the umbrella term 'behavioural and psychological symptoms of dementia' or 'BPSD' is often used. BPSD has been accepted to describe symptoms of disturbed perception, thought content, mood or actions that frequently occur in people with dementia. Whilst this might be a convenient short hand, BPSD must not be mistaken for another diagnosis on top of a dementia. Instead, it is frequently a communication that needs to be understood.

At some stage in their illness, up to 90% of people with dementia will experience behavioural or psychological challenges. Symptoms can arise at any stage of a person's illness, and multiple symptoms often occur at the same time and on a recurring basis.

Importantly, nearly two-thirds of people with dementia living in care homes experience these symptoms. The most obvious to those looking after a resident are behaviours such as agitation, aggression, shouting and wandering, but there can also be personal, internal experiences such as depression, delusions or hallucinations which are not so noticeable, but are equally as important (Box 8.1).

ABC of Dementia, First Edition. Edited by Bernard Coope and Felicity Richards.
© 2014 John Wiley & Sons, Ltd. Published 2014 by John Wiley & Sons, Ltd.

Box 8.1 Examples of behavioural and psychological symptoms of dementia

Behavioural symptoms	Psychological symptoms
<ul><li>Screaming</li><li>Shouting</li><li>Swearing</li><li>Restlessness</li><li>Agitation and physical aggression</li><li>Walking without purpose</li><li>Sexual disinhibition</li><li>Hoarding</li><li>Searching or following</li></ul>	<ul><li>Mood disturbance – depression, elation</li><li>Anxiety symptoms</li><li>Perceptual abnormalities – hallucinations Delusional beliefs</li></ul>

Impact on carers and prediction of institutionalisation

Behavioural and psychological changes can affect not only a person with dementia but also everyone involved in their care and treatment.

The symptoms can cause distress to the individual, and when a person retains a certain amount of insight into their losses there is the potential for more feelings of desperation, anger and frustration. It is important to add that not all behavioural symptoms cause distress to the person with dementia, but rather cause 'difficulties' for those around them – for example, repetitive shouting, walking without a purpose or displaying attachment behaviour, and therefore should not be considered 'symptoms that need treatment', rather understanding. Sexual behaviour is another example. It may be unacceptable to other residents in a care setting, but not to the individual. It is in a person's best interests therefore to acknowledge this behaviour, and plan care appropriately.

However, the emergence of behavioural and psychological features add considerably to the anxieties experienced by family and professional carers, who understandably can find the changes in their relative very difficult to adjust to – especially if those behaviours put the individual or others at risk. A sense that the essence of their loved one has been lost prevails, as behaviours exhibited can be radically different to pre-morbid behaviour and personality and out of character.

Indeed, the frequency of behavioural disturbances has been identified as the strongest predictor of caregiver stress and plays a significant role in the decision to institutionalise a person with dementia.

Legal framework

Many people with dementia experiencing behavioural and psychological change do not have the mental capacity to make informed decisions about their treatment and management. Management not only includes medication for physical or mental health issues, but general hands-on care such as washing, dressing, nutritional needs and end-of-life issues.

Health care professionals are often in the best position to assess capacity for certain decisions under the Mental Capacity Act 2005 (Box 8.2, see Chapter 12 for more details). Capacity should be presumed, until proven otherwise. A capacity assessment is important in order to find out if persons with dementia and BPSD have an understanding of the risks involved with their behaviour, for example, not accepting assistance with hands-on personal care, refusal of medication or not accepting that their care needs now require them to be residents in a care-home setting.

If a person is in a care home, it is also the care home's responsibility to construct a clear individualised care plan including outlining a person's care needs, which can include discussions and shared-care decisions regarding basic human needs such as maintaining cleanliness, nutrition and dignity. All decisions should be made in the person's best interests, include any Advance Statement, and involve relatives/informal carers, especially if an LPA Lasting Power of Attorney or COP Court of Protection is held.

Box 8.2 **Functional test of capacity**

Can the person …
… **understand** the information relevant to the decision?
… **retain** that information?
… **weigh** that information as part of a process of making a decision?
… **communicate** his/her decision (talking, sign language or other means)?
Clear record of the test for capacity and documentation of the process is good practice.

There will be times when decisions about deprivation of liberty need to be assessed. For example, a person may be agitated, anxious and constantly trying to abscond from a care environment to return to their home or childhood home. Under such circumstances, an application can be made to the local authority for a Deprivation of Liberty Safeguards (DoLS) assessment so that treatment and care can be provided in the person's best interests.

Assessment and management of BPSD

The assessment and management of behavioural and psychological symptoms in an individual with dementia is a dynamic and continuous process of proactively assessing for potential problems, understanding patterns of symptoms and deciding on the most appropriate course of action to take. Quite often, elements of this process will occur in conjunction with each other.

The Alzheimer's Society has produced a best practice guide for health and social care professionals who are involved in the treatment and care of people with BPSD. The recommended approach involves the process of actively working to 'prevent' the emergence or escalation of BPSD, adopting 'watchful waiting' if this does occur, and only after this considering 'specific interventions'.

Prevention

A number of simple approaches that can help reduce the chance of BPSD developing are recommended. This information will help inform an effective care plan for the person with dementia (see Box 8.3).

Box 8.3 **Prevention of BPSD**

(i) Understanding of dementia
(ii) Medical review
(iii) Recognition of triggers and early signs
(iv) Pharmacological treatments
(v) Physical environment

Understanding of dementia

No two people are the same. No two dementias are the same. We are all affected differently. There are many types of dementia, all with varying presentations. We need to recognise this, understand an individual's dementia, and also understand the individual.

Being aware of and understanding the needs of a person with dementia can help prevent challenging behaviours and psychological symptoms. There are frequently social and environmental triggers associated with symptoms. Behaviours often have specific meaning for the person with dementia and may be a way of communicating their needs. For example, agitation may arise from boredom or a recent change in routine or environment. Simple adjustments to social interactions and environment can make a significant difference to the person's quality of life and that of their carer(s). It is therefore vital that health professionals and carers seek to understand the needs of a person with dementia – the aim here is to improve quality of life, not 'treat'.

The approach of 'person-centred care' is very helpful. As outlined in Chapter 7, skilled person-centred care and support can reduce the occurrence or escalation of problems into BPSD. This approach is based on understanding the person's history and experiences (their work, life, hobbies, family, environment and religious beliefs), their likes and dislikes and taking their perspective into account. A simple clinical care plan (for simple non-drug treatments) can be designed around the person's needs, abilities and interests.

Medical review

If in doubt, take a history, and thoroughly assess. A medical review by a general practitioner (GP) is essential to detect any general health problems, but also recognise change. For example, pain is identified as a major trigger for agitation and aggression, and infections can cause a broad range of symptoms. Identifying the need for analgesia or antibiotic treatment at an early stage can be a useful approach in preventing or managing behavioural disturbance, and can help focus an assessment and put treatments in place early. A medication review can minimise potential drug interactions, and discontinue medications that could affect cognitive functioning (see Chapter 5). Think of simple treatable causes first – dehydration, infection, pain, constipation, medication interactions and the environment.

Recognition of triggers and early signs

Recognition of triggers and early signs can help in the prevention of symptoms through the implementation of simple measures. Physical signs include pain, discomfort, malnourishment, dehydration and physical illness. Psychological signs include stress, boredom, irritability, mood disturbance, suspiciousness, increased levels of distress, misidentification syndrome and hallucinations. Time of day may be a trigger, for example, increasing confusion towards the end of the day may be due to the 'sundowning' effect of changes in circadian rhythms. It is also important to be alert to signs of abuse or neglect. Triggers can also include help with personal interventions, having a new carer, changes in environment, that is, admission to hospital, or a move to a different care home.

The sudden emergence of BPSD often has a physical trigger, for example, delirium or cerebrovascular event. Longer onset emergence can be linked to depression. Often, there isn't a simple 'cause' or single trigger that is identifiable.

Pharmacological treatments

Acetylcholinesterase inhibitors (donepezil, rivastigmine, galantamine) and memantine are licensed for mild to moderate and moderate-to-severe Alzheimer's disease, respectively, not frontotemporal or vascular dementia. There is some evidence that both groups may delay the onset of BPSD, providing additional benefit to using these treatment options.

Physical environment

It is important to consider the person's environment and how it might affect them. Optimizing vision and hearing so that an individual can appreciate the physical surrounds and the presence of company is crucial in preventing distress and other associated symptoms such as shouting. Visual correction can help prevent falls. Consider whether glasses are the person's own and are clean. Check that hearing aids are turned on and working properly.

Consider whether the individual is mobile, in a wheelchair or being nursed in bed. Determine whether the person is able to move about freely if mobile and if assistive technology can be used to improve freedom or safety. If nursed in a bed, consider whether the person is comfortable and not in pain, for example, from pressure sores.

Consider the nature of activity in the environment. Is there sufficient opportunity for meaningful social interaction and other activities such as music or television programmes that the person can relate to, and enjoy? And, if not, why not?

Watchful waiting

Unless there is extreme distress or risk, it is recommended that first-line interventions (as described earlier), ongoing assessment and watchful waiting are tried with all people. Behavioural and psychological symptoms in dementia often disappear over 4 weeks without the need for medication. It is important to identify and address any triggers or unmet needs that may have caused the symptoms. Simple changes in treatment and care can avoid the use of sedating medication and antipsychotic drugs in people with dementia.

Consulting with family

It is essential to discuss the person's symptoms and possible treatments with their family or carer, and this is clearly outlined in the Mental Capacity Act 2005 Code of Practice. Family and carers may be able to shed light on the reasons for their symptoms and ways to engage their relative in activities.

As mentioned previously, it is likely that the person experiencing BPSD has lost the capacity to make decisions about treatment and management. Discussing treatment options in order to make shared decisions in a person's best interests is an essential part of care, especially if considering antipsychotics – indeed, discussions with family/carers are recommended by NICE (see Box 8.5).

Soothing and creative therapies

These can include aromatherapy, massage, having one's hair brushed or a manicure. Music can help improve a person's mood. Singing and dancing can energise people and lift spirits. See also Box 8.4.

Specific interventions

Specific psychological and pharmacological approaches are recommended if symptoms have not spontaneously resolved or improved with first-line interventions and watchful waiting, i.e., daily brief 1 : 1 conversation or personalised activities, for example, looking at pictures from their past can help engage people and improve symptoms. Exercise, for example, gentle stretching can help improve physical well-being, cognition and mood.

Box 8.4 **Simple non-drug treatments and sleep hygiene**

Simple non-drug treatments	Sleep hygiene
Developing a life story book	Consider reducing daytime napping
Frequent short conversations (up to 30 seconds)	Consider increasing activities during the day
Using personal care as an opportunity for positive social interaction	Agreeing to realistic expectations for sleep duration

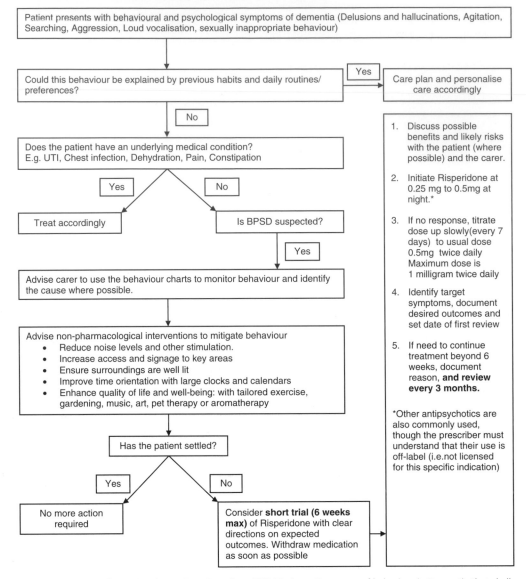

Guidelines for the management of behavioural and psychological symptoms in patients with Dementia (BPSD) in Primary Care/ Care Homes
NB: This flow chart does not applyin Palliative care patients

Patient presents with behavioural and psychological symptoms of dementia (Delusions and hallucinations, Agitation, Searching, Aggression, Loud vocalisation, sexually inappropriate behaviour)

Could this behaviour be explained by previous habits and daily routines/ preferences?

Yes → Care plan and personalise care accordingly

No

Does the patient have an underlying medical condition? E.g. UTI, Chest infection, Dehydration, Pain, Constipation

Yes → Treat accordingly

No → Is BPSD suspected?

Yes

Advise carer to use the behaviour charts to monitor behaviour and identify the cause where possible.

Advise non-pharmacological interventions to mitigate behaviour
- Reduce noise levels and other stimulation.
- Increase access and signage to key areas
- Ensure surroundings are well lit
- Improve time orientation with large clocks and calendars
- Enhance quality of life and well-being: with tailored exercise, gardening, music, art, pet therapy or aromatherapy

Has the patient settled?

Yes → No more action required

No → Consider **short trial (6 weeks max)** of Risperidone with clear directions on expected outcomes. Withdraw medication as soon as possible

1. Discuss possible benefits and likely risks with the patient (where possible) and the carer.

2. Initiate Risperidone at 0.25 mg to 0.5mg at night.*

3. If no response, titrate dose up slowly(every 7 days) to usual dose 0.5mg twice daily Maximum dose is 1 milligram twice daily

4. Identify target symptoms, document desired outcomes and set date of first review

5. If need to continue treatment beyond 6 weeks, document reason, **and review every 3 months.**

*Other antipsychotics are also commonly used, though the prescriber must understand that their use is off-label (i.e.not licensed for this specific indication)

Figure 8.1 Guidelines for management of BPSD in Primary Care. Data from NHS Medway, *Treatment of behaviour in Dementia that challenges.'*

Pharmacological treatments

Certain medications can be utilized, if appropriate. Before commencing medications, however, consider whether the symptoms are severe and persistent enough, are affecting the person's life in a detrimental way (rather than the lives of others around them) and, importantly, whether other aspects have been considered such as physical health, the environment and quality of care. Always remember the aim of an intervention is to improve a person's quality of life.

If a care home is not focused on person-centred dementia care, has limited understanding of the person with dementia and is clearly not meeting that individual's needs, it may be more appropriate to move the person to a more suitable placement, rather than use antipsychotic or sedating medication.

Specific medications

Antipsychotics can be used but NICE guidance should be followed (see Box 8.5). The only licensed antipsychotic for use in BPSD is risperidone, but other antipsychotics are commonly used. Always start at the lowest dose (i.e risperidone 0.25 mg nocte) and titrate slowly if necessary. NICE has produced clinical criteria for the use of antipsychotic medication for non-cognitive symptoms, behaviour that challenges and behaviour control.

Box 8.5 **NICE guidelines on the prescribing of antipsychotics in dementia**

1 There should be a full discussion with the person with dementia and/or carers about possible benefits and risks of treatment.
2 Cerebrovascular risk factors should be assessed and possible increased risk of stroke/transient ischaemic attack (TIA) and possible adverse effects on cognition discussed.
3 Changes in cognition should be assessed and recorded at regular intervals.
4 Target symptoms should be identified, quantified and documented.
5 Changes in target symptoms should be assessed and recorded at regular intervals.
6 The effect of comorbid conditions, such as depression, should be considered before offering an antipsychotic.
7 Choice of antipsychotic should be made after an individual risk–benefit analysis.
8 Dose should be low initially and then titrated upwards if needed.
9 Treatment to be time limited and regularly reviewed (every 3 months or according to clinical need).

There is no evidence for the use of benzodiazepines, which can lead to oversedation, falls, tolerability and withdrawal. Acetylcholinesterase inhibitors can delay the onset of BPSD, but can also increase hyperarousal and irritability in those suffering from behavioural changes, and are often discontinued for this reason. Memantine can be used in moderate/severe dementia.

BPSD is commonly managed in primary care by a person's GP. **A helpful approach for primary care and care homes is outlined in Figure** 8.1. A number of people who are greatly affected by behavioural challenges are referred to secondary mental health services for involvement of a community psychiatric nurse, or nursing home liaison service if commissioned. Medication can be prescribed either in primary or secondary care, treatment should be time limited, and regularly reviewed every three months. See Box 8.6. Some people may require long-term use of antipsychotic treatment to improve their quality of life and prevent ongoing distress.

Box 8.6 **General guidance for discontinuing/withdrawing antipsychotic medication**

1 Halve the dose for 1 week and if there are no emerging symptoms, stop the drug.
2 Review after 1 week.
3 If symptoms re-emerge, reintroduce the drug at the starting dose. BPSD can persist and treatment with anti-psychotics may be needed longer term, but should be reviewed on a 3-monthly basis.

Conclusion

We must not forget that our psychological variations and behaviours are not an illness, but, in the context of a dementia, can lead to challenges for the patient, family and care environment. Acknowledging the person with dementia as an individual, and using a person-centred approach is the most important step in preventing the occurrence or escalation of BPSD. Frequently, behavioural changes are a communication from the person with dementia. Antipsychotic medication has a small role to play, but careful consideration should be made regarding the benefits versus risks of these medications in relieving some of the distress experienced by those affected.

Case study applying the person-centred approach as used by a Nursing Home In-reach Team

Mrs X has a diagnosis of vascular dementia. She was referred to the In-Reach Team by the community mental health team because of reported increased agitation, restlessness and resistance to personal care. She had been admitted to the care home 5 months before the referral following a severe stroke and at the time her prognosis had not been good. She had improved physically; however, staff were finding her behaviour difficult to manage and initially requested that medication be prescribed to settle her.

Physical investigations revealed that Mrs X had a urinary tract infection (UTI) and indeed records showed that she was prone to UTIs and became significantly more confused when infection was present. Staff were advised to screen for a UTI proactively. Analgesia was also looked at and staff were advised to ensure regular pain relief was given as Mrs X suffers from scoliosis and pain increases her agitation and impacts upon compliance with personal care.

Sensory impairment was noted and following audiology input hearing aids were provided and found to make a huge difference to communication. Mrs X was able to understand and express herself clearly, reducing the risk of misinterpretation and the potential for angry outbursts, especially around personal care. Staff also observed that she was functioning at a higher level cognitively than assumed before sensory impairment being fully assessed.

Further assessment of mobility had shown that Mrs X could weight bear and she was able to sit in a chair. Sitting in a chair provided much more stimulation and the opportunity to socialise in communal areas and enjoy meals, thereby improving dietary/fluid intake. Staff members were encouraged to take positive risks and to accept that normal life comes with a certain amount of acceptable risk. They were also supported with care plans for each identified need.

Staff training was provided around person-centred care (Kitwood and Brooker models) to build understanding and empathy around presenting behaviours. Staff members were presented with information about Mrs X's biography including traumatic bereavements she suffered and her strong religious beliefs, aiding staff to understand that she may sometimes relive traumatic events and that she finds personal care difficult to accept as she had always managed this herself.

Occupation and stimulation were addressed and a rummage box provided Mrs X with a focus when staff members were not able to spend time with her. She was also noted to enjoy group reminiscence and music. Other ideas were looking at photos and pictures; utilising sensory items, aromatherapy, pet therapy and meaningful occupation which involved folding towels and cleaning items.

Family members were also requested to be involved. They brought in new clothes for Mrs X rather than night attire only, and brought in items from home to personalise her bedroom, providing a much more pleasant environment and encouraging staff to see her as a person with a rich history and personal preferences. The staff learnt that Mrs X had always been an extrovert and needed regular social contact to prevent loneliness and lowness of mood.

There was a need in the home to restore personhood and for people to start relating to Mrs X rather than seeing her as ill and a body in a bed. Overall, the culture in the home had been addressed and input was provided to support the home with the adjustments that were needed to improve quality of life not only for Mrs X but for other residents and care staff as well.

Further reading

Alzheimer's Society: *Best Practice Guide for Health and Social Care Professionals. Optimising Treatment and Care for People with Behavioural and Psychological Symptoms of Dementia*. Advisory group co-chaired by Prof. Alistair Burns and Prof. Clive Ballard.

Institute for Innovation and Improvement, Dementia Action Alliance, Department of Health. *The Right Prescription – A Call to Action for Junior Doctors on the Use of Antipsychotic Drugs for People with Dementia*.

CHAPTER 9

Dementia in Younger People

Peter Bentham

Birmingham Memory Assessment and Rare Dementia Services, Birmingham, UK

> **OVERVIEW**
> - There are over 15,000 younger people with dementia in the UK.
> - Compared to older people, there is marked aetiological heterogeneity.
> - Some causes of dementia, although rare, are potentially reversible.
> - The needs of younger people with dementia cannot be adequately met by older adult services.
> - Specialist provision with clear care pathways is required.

Epidemiology

Owing to methodological complexities, no epidemiological studies have been conducted to ascertain the prevalence of dementia in young adults. In 2005, based on two clinical studies, it was estimated that just over 15,000 adults aged under 65 years in the UK had dementia. These numbers are predicted to slowly rise to over 17,000 by 2021. It is however generally recognised that these numbers are substantial underestimates, and the true figure could be up to three times higher. The risk of early-onset dementia increases with age but in contrast to older people, it is more common in males (Table 9.1). It may also be more common in black and ethnic minority groups, where 6.1% of dementia is early onset, compared with 2.2% of the total dementia population. The low relative prevalence of early onset dementia (85/100,000), in comparison with functional disorders causing cognitive impairment in younger people such as schizophrenia (4/1000), makes diagnosis particularly challenging.

Diagnosis

The vast majority of dementia in older people can be accounted for by three pathologies: Alzheimer's disease (AD), cerebrovascular disease and Lewy body disease. The situation in younger adults is far more complex. Whilst AD remains the commonest cause, it probably accounts for less than one-half of the diagnoses, and over 30% of cases are due to frontotemporal dementia (FTD) or other rare disorders (Figure 9.1).

ABC of Dementia, First Edition. Edited by Bernard Coope and Felicity Richards.
© 2014 John Wiley & Sons, Ltd. Published 2014 by John Wiley & Sons, Ltd.

Table 9.1 Prevalence of early onset dementia per 100,000 UK population.

Age	F	M	Total
30–34	9.5	8.9	9.4
35–39	9.3	6.3	7.7
40–44	19.6	8.1	14.0
45–49	27.3	31.8	30.4
50–54	55.1	62.7	58.3
55–59	97.1	179.5	136.8
60–64	118.0	198.9	155.7
45–64	66.2	99.5	84.7

Knapp et al. (2007). Reproduced by permission of the Alzheimer's Society.

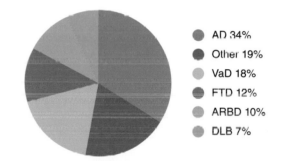

- AD 34%
- Other 19%
- VaD 18%
- FTD 12%
- ARBD 10%
- DLB 7%

Figure 9.1 Early-onset dementia diagnostic subtypes. .Harvey et al. (2003). Reproduced with permission from BMJ Publishing Group Ltd.

Accurate diagnosis of dementia in younger people is difficult, with incorrect or uncertain diagnoses reported in 30–50% cases. Service users frequently report delays in diagnosis and in being 'pushed from pillar to post' in the process (Williams et al., 1999). Diagnosis is particularly difficult in people with a history of functional psychiatric disorder or learning disability and in those from ethnic minority groups, where cultural and linguistic influences on cognitive test performance make interpretation difficult. It is particularly important that functional psychiatric disorders, such as depression, and drugs are excluded, as they are far more common causes of cognitive impairment in younger adults than true dementia. Table 9.2 summarises aetiological subtypes of dementia encountered in younger people based on their earliest or most prominent clinical manifestations.

Although less than 1% of true dementia may be partly or fully reversible (Box 9.1), nearly all of these cases occur in younger

Table 9.2 Causes of dementia in younger people.

Clinical presentation	Clinical features	Disorders
Amnestic Dementia	Inability to learn and retain new information	• Alzheimer's disease • WKS
Dysphasic dementia	Problems with combinations of semantic, phonemic and syntactical aspects of speech and language	• Progressive aphasias • Alzheimer's disease • Vascular dementia • CBS/PSP • SOL • CJD
Subcortical dementia	Impaired attentional control Executive dysfunction Cognitive slowing Neurological deficits	• Vascular dementia • Parkinsonian dementia • HIV dementia • Hydrocephalus • Multiple sclerosis • Huntington's disease
Parkinsonian dementia	Subcortical pattern of cognitive impairment Extrapyramidal neurological deficit	• PDD/DLB • Vascular dementia • CBS/PSP/MSA • Huntington's disease • FTDP-17 • Wilson's disease • CJD
Psychiatric dementia	Behavioural change, hallucinations and mood disorder	• bvFTD • DLB • Vascular dementia • Neurosyphilis • Variant CJD • LE
Dyspraxic dementia	Inability to perform learnt patterns of motor function including gait disturbance	• Alzheimer's disease • CBS • Vascular dementia • Hydrocephalus • Primary progressive aphasia • CJD
Jerky or tremulous dementia	Chorea Tremor Jerks	• Huntington's disease • SCA • DRPLA • Neuroacanthocytosis • Parkinsonian dementias • SCA • Ataxic dementias • Myoclonic dementias
Ataxic dementia	Incoordination and gait disturbance	• WKS • Vascular dementia • Multiple sclerosis • SCA • CTE • LE • CJD
Myoclonic dementias	Myoclonic jerks	• Degenerative (DLB, CBS) • Infectious (CJD) • Autoimmune (LE) • Metabolic (Kuf's) • Mitochondrial (MELAS)
Fluctuating dementia	Features of delirium	• Dementia + delirium • DLB • Vascular dementia • Subdural/SOL • LE • CJD
Familial dementia	Familial aggregation, particularly at younger age	• AD • FTD • CADASIL • HD • SCA • Leukodystrophy
Rapidly progressive dementia	Progression to death within few months to 3–4 years	• CJD • Neurodegenerative (FTD–ALS) • Autoimmune (vasculitis) • Neoplastic (lymphoma) • Other infectious (HIV) • Toxic (lead) • Metabolic (Kuf's)

WKS, Wernike–Korsakoff syndrome; CBS, corticobasal syndrome; PSP, progressive supranuclear palsy; SOL, space-occupying lesion; CJD, Creutzfeld–Jacob disease; HIV, human immunodeficiency virus; PDD, Parkinson's disease dementia; DLB, dementia with Lewy bodies; MSA, multi-system atrophy; FTDP-17, frontotemporal dementia linked to chromosome 17; bvFTD, behavioural variant frontotemporal dementia; LE, limbic encephalopathy; SCA, spino-cerebellar ataxia; DRPLA, dentato rubro pallido lysurian atrophy; CTE, chronic traumatic encephalopathy; MELAS, mitochondrial encephalomyopathy with lactic acidosis and stroke-like episodes; ALS, amyotrophic lateral sclerosis.

adults (Clarfield, 2003). Consequently, it is essential that younger people with dementia are thoroughly investigated by specialist services, with structural neuroimaging, preferably magnetic resonance imaging (MRI), being a mandatory requirement. Multiprofessional input into the diagnostic process is essential, and may require the coordinated efforts of psychiatrists, neurologists, clinical psychologists, neuroradiologists, and geneticists.

Aetiological subtypes

Alzheimer's disease: AD, as in older people, usually presents with insidious onset, progressive impairment of memory for recent events, with particular difficulty in semantic encoding and delayed recall. It may, however, present atypically as posterior cortical atrophy with disturbed visuospatial function (see Chapter 2). Some AD patients also present with prominent language disturbance or executive dysfunction.

Frontotemporal Dementia: FTD can be broadly divided into two clinical presentations, behavioural and dysphasic. Behavioural variant FTD is characterised by insidious-onset progressive change in personality and behaviour (Box 9.2). It is important to confirm that there is neuroimaging evidence of frontal or temporal atrophy or similarly located metabolic or blood flow abnormalities, as those who lack these features tend to deteriorate little and may have a different disorder. In the UK, around 40% of cases have a positive family history, and a significant proportion of these will have mutations in the genes for tau or progranulin, or the *C9ORF72* hexanucleotide repeat, which is also associated with amyotrophic lateral sclerosis.

In progressive aphasias, there is gradual onset, deteriorating language function, which is the predominant symptom during the initial phase of the illness. There are broadly three types: semantic dementia, progressive non-fluent aphasia and logopenic aphasia (Table 9.3).

Dementias of other aetiology: Dementias occurring in parkinsonism usually have a subcortical pattern of cognitive impairment, as classically described in progressive supranuclear palsy (PSP). Marked visuoperceptual impairment, fluctuation and recurrent visual hallucinations suggest dementia with Lewy bodies, whereas prominent apraxia and asymmetric rigidity are features of corticobasal syndrome. Those with multisystem atrophy, however, rarely develop more severe dementia. Human immunodeficiency virus (HIV)-associated dementia also has a subcortical pattern, often with marked slowing of information processing and motor clumsiness. Gait dyspraxia should suggest hydrocephalus, particularly if there is early urinary incontinence.

Genetics: Although the vast majority of dementia in younger people occurs sporadically, some cases are due to gene mutations. This may be suggested by the atypical nature of the symptoms such as chorea in Huntington's disease (HD), or a very early age of onset. Sometimes, MRI scan appearances may suggest a genetic aetiology with marked typical white matter abnormalities occurring in cerebral autosomal-dominant arteriopathy with subcortical infarcts and leukoencephalopathy (CADASIL) and leukodystrophies. However, occasionally, typical clinical presentations such as AD occurring in late middle age can be due

Table 9.3 Progressive aphasias.

	Semantic	Non-fluent	Logopenic
Clinical features	Fluent speech Anomia Impaired single-word comprehension Surface dyslexia Spared repetition	Effortful, agrammatic speech Apraxia of speech Impaired syntactical comprehension Preserved object knowledge	Slow speech Word finding pauses Impaired sentence repetition and comprehension Reduced word span Preserved object knowledge
Imaging abnormalities	Left anterior temporal	Left posterior frontal and insular	Left posterior temporal and inferior parietal lobule
Pathology	TDP-43	Tauopathy	AD type

Gorno-tempini et al. (2011). Reproduced by permission of Wolters Kluwer Health.

to dominantly inherited mutations, usually in the presenilin 1 (PS1) or less commonly amyloid precursor protein (APP) genes. Conversely, very early-onset FTD, in the absence of a family history, is rarely found to be due to a mutation. It is therefore important to take a careful family history, including first- and second-degree relatives, in all cases of dementia occurring in younger people.

Patients with rapidly progressive dementia require urgent neurological investigation as do those with early myoclonus or seizures, as the aetiology is often non-neurodegenerative. Whilst conditions like Creutzfeldt–Jakob (CJD) continue to have a very poor prognosis, others such as some forms of limbic encephalopathy, which may also have prominent psychiatric symptomatology, respond well to immunological therapy.

Pharmacological treatment

Whilst younger people with AD can be treated in much the same way as older people with the same disorder, perhaps with less risk, the findings from AD studies cannot simply be applied to other diagnoses. Patients with FTD do not respond to cholinesterase inhibitors, which indeed may worsen their symptoms. They are particularly sensitive to the side effects of antipsychotic drugs but some aspects of their behaviour may benefit from treatment with trazodone.

Comprehensive assessment and support

Accurate diagnosis alone is insufficient. Younger people with dementia, their families and supporters require a comprehensive, multidisciplinary review of their needs followed by an individualised, age-appropriate care plan. These needs are seldom adequately met by conventional social care services, which are designed for frail older people. In particular, day care, respite and residential facilities for the elderly tend to be ill suited to the needs of younger people. Direct Payments, used to fund personalised support, is a good, flexible method of overcoming some of these limitations.

Information needs

Younger people with dementia and their families frequently report a lack of adequate information and counselling, particularly around the time of diagnosis. Information about the diagnosis and its implications in terms of treatment and prognosis must be given in a timely, user-friendly and sensitive format. Whilst information on AD abounds, it may be very difficult to access in an easily digestible form for some of the rarer conditions. Education programmes and telephone helplines can be useful sources of information.

Undergoing assessment for possible dementia is daunting, frightening and in some ways disadvantageous. Preassessment counselling is essential in enabling people to prepare for and give informed consent to an assessment.

Developing dementia at a young age is usually financially disastrous for the individual and the family. This situation is compounded by the complex nature of the benefits system. Impartial advice and information provided by a specialist social worker or benefits advisor can be invaluable.

Social needs

The majority of younger people with dementia are in paid employment at the time of onset and, indeed, occupational dysfunction is a common presenting feature of dementia in younger people. Risk assessment is of pivotal importance and may require a workplace occupational therapy assessment. It is not unusual for younger people with dementia to be made redundant or be dismissed from work. Employers should be encouraged to recognise dementia as a reason for early retirement so that pension rights and other benefits are not affected. Furthermore, some younger people with dementia wish to remain in employment, and efforts should be made to encourage employers to make reasonable workplace adjustments to accommodate disabilities and maximise strengths. It is quite common for younger people with dementia to be drivers. Where doubt remains about driving ability, particularly in atypical presentations, referral to a Regional Driving Assessment Centre will usually provide clarity.

Carer and family needs

Caring for a younger person with dementia is a major source of stress and burden, both known important risk factors for institutionalisation. Approximately one-half of carers of younger people with dementia have psychiatric morbidity, usually anxiety or depression. Carers have a legal right to have their own needs assessed, but it is also important to recognise and meet the needs of the wider family. Children and adolescents, who may also be carers, are also adversely affected and can sometimes require help from children's services. Timely input from an experienced specialist community mental health or Admiral Nurse is particularly valued by families, especially when this support can be provided throughout the illness. Marked disruption in family dynamics, however,

may require specialised input from family therapy services. Family members frequently overestimate their risk of inheriting dementia and can be reassured by accurate information. Additional complications, however, do arise for families when an inherited disorder is suspected, requiring liaison with genetic services and the provision of counselling and possible genetic testing.

Physical needs

Some forms of early-onset dementia are associated with an increased risk of choking, either as a result of abnormal eating behaviour or neurological dysfunction. Here, assessment by a speech and language therapist is an important part of the risk assessment. They will also be able to advise on management of dysphasia, which can be a major frustration to both patient and carer, increasing the risk of behavioural disturbance. Falls are particularly problematic in conditions such as HD and PSP, requiring input from physiotherapy. Dietary advice is important in conditions resulting in excessive weight loss (HD) or gain (FTD).

Service development

For successful, sustained service development, specific commissioning arrangements based on local need are required, with individuals identified at both a purchaser and provider level with responsibility for the service. There must be strong clinical leadership from well-motivated, experienced, specialists with dedicated clinical time. For populations of 500,000 and above, a dedicated multidisciplinary team is justified. Younger people and their families should be involved as partners in service development, and there must also be close collaboration with other services, with clear but flexible demarcation of responsibilities. Initial development should concentrate on diagnosis and community-based support.

Institutionalisation risk appears disproportionately high in younger people with dementia, with up to 30% residing in some form of care. It has been estimated that approximately 15 residential, nursing or long-stay places are required for every 100,000 people at risk (Harvey et al., 2003). Although institutional care can be delayed and sometimes avoided by good community care, specialist long-stay provision remains essential, because younger, physically robust patients with dementia generally do not mix well with their frail, older counterparts. Psychiatric admission is best avoided, as the needs of younger people with dementia cannot usually be adequately met on either older adult or general-adult wards.

Box 9.1 Reversible causes of dementia

- Drugs (e.g. valproate)
- Infection (e.g. HIV)
- Autoimmune (e.g. anti-voltage-gated potassium channel (VGKC) antibodies)
- Space-occupying lesion (e.g. hydrocephalus)
- Nutritional deficiency (e.g. B12)
- Metabolic (e.g. Wilson's disease)
- Functional mental disorder (e.g. depression)

Box 9.2 **Clinical features of behavioural variant frontotemporal dementia**

- Early behavioural disinhibition
- Early apathy or inertia
- Early loss of sympathy or empathy
- Early perseverative, stereotyped, compulsive or ritualistic behaviour
- Hyperorality and dietary changes
- Executive deficits predominate over memory and visuospatial problems

Rascovsky et al. (2011). Reproduced with permission from Oxford University Press.

Services for younger people with dementia should be based on a philosophy of person- and family-centred care, with clear care pathways, and capable of meeting a person and the family's needs at all stages of the illness so that they are no longer 'pushed from pillar to post'.

References

Clarfield AM. The decreasing prevalence of reversible dementias: an updated meta-analysis. *Arch Int Med* 2003; **16**:2219–2229.

Gorno-tempini ML, Hillis AE, Weintraub S et al. Classification of primary progressive aphasias. *Neurology* 2011; **76**:1006–1014.

Harvey RJ, Skelton-Robinson M, Rossor MN. The prevalence and causes of dementia in people under the age of 65 years. *J Neurol Neurosurg Psych* 2003 September; **74**(9):1206–1209.

Knapp M, Prince M, Albanese E et al. *Dementia UK: The Full Report.* Alzheimer's Society: London, 2007.

Rascovsky K, Hodges JR, Knopman D, et al. Sensitivity of revised diagnostic criteria for the behavioural variant of frontotemporal dementia. *Brain* 2011; **134**:2456–2477.

Williams T, Cameron I, Deardon T, et al. *From Pillar to Post: Early Onset Dementia in Leeds: Prevalence, Experience and Service Needs.* Leeds Health Authority: Leeds, 1999.

CHAPTER 10

Dementia in Primary Care

Simon Rumley

Aylmer Lodge Cookley Partnership, Kidderminster, Worcestershire, UK

OVERVIEW

- Dementia is an area of growing importance for primary care.
- Incidence and prevalence of dementia are increasing in line with an ageing population.
- Primary care teams have a vital role to play in enabling patients with dementia to live well.
- The future role of the primary care team is likely to further develop with a flexible approach to partnership working.

Introduction

This chapter examines the role of the primary care team in the management of patients with dementia. Traditional interventions such as medication play a limited role. Instead, management focuses on enabling the patient with dementia to live to the maximum of his or her potential. To achieve this, the primary care team must play its role as part of a wide network of individuals and organisations, all working towards this aim.

Primary care is well placed for this task. The general practitioner (GP) may already have an established relationship with the patient and other members of the family and will have a good understanding of the current health status and previous history. The patient's journey, from diagnosis to end of life, will often be shared with the GP.

Prevalence of dementia

The percentage of people with dementia who have received a diagnosis in the UK increased from 43.3% in 2011 to 46% in 2012. This illustrates what is referred to as the 'dementia gap', that is, the differential between expected and recorded diagnoses of the condition. This percentage varies considerably from area to area.

Local prevalence will be affected by demographic features, including the cultural and ethnic make-up of each practice population. Incidence and prevalence will continue to increase because of the increasing proportion of older adults in the population.

Primary care will be required to play a key role in managing these increasing numbers.

Closing the dementia gap – working towards earlier diagnosis

The above-mentioned figures suggest that less than half of the people with dementia in the UK have been given a diagnosis of dementia. The estimated prevalence figure has a large margin of error, being based on census figures rather than diagnostic criteria, but there is widespread acceptance that a large cohort of undiagnosed individuals exists in the UK.

Although there may be some benefit in earlier pharmacological treatment to treat symptoms arising from dementia, the main advantages in an earlier diagnosis lie in enabling the patient with dementia, together with family and carers, to come to terms with the condition and to plan for the future, while the patient still has the capacity to do so. This opportunity can be formalised by engaging in the process known as advance decision planning. For further information, see Chapter 12.

Some authorities support formal screening for dementia. An example of this approach would be testing the cognitive function of individuals at a younger age than the expected onset of dementia. This would aim to pick up early signs of cognitive decline. However, screening for dementia does not fulfil standard criteria. Having identified an individual at an earlier stage of the disease process, a positive intervention which will alter the course of the disease needs to be identified, and such an intervention is yet to be demonstrated.

Box 10.1 Groups of patients to consider when undertaking a case-finding search for dementia

- Patients over the age of 75
- Patients with a read code of, for example, memory loss, forgetfulness, confusion
- Patients taking donepezil, galantamine, rivastigmine (the acetylcholinesterase inhibitors) and memantine, not yet on the Quality and Outcomes Framework (QOF) register
- Patients over 60 on anti-psychotic medication
- Patients with learning difficulties or Down's syndrome over the age of 40

ABC of Dementia, First Edition. Edited by Bernard Coope and Felicity Richards.
© 2014 John Wiley & Sons, Ltd. Published 2014 by John Wiley & Sons, Ltd.

- Younger patients who may be developing young-onset dementia
- Patients with a history of Parkinson's disease, stroke, major head injury or chronic alcohol problems over the age of 60
- Patients permanently residing in care homes

Case finding may be a more appropriate approach. This involves searching for patients with clinical features of dementia who have not been identified and diagnosed with the condition. Possible groups of patients to focus on when conducting such a search are included in Box 10.1.

Prevention

It would seem logical and good practice to plan interventions as early as possible in the course of dementia, in order to prevent or delay the onset of the condition. This area is currently generating a great deal of interest. As yet, however, there is no definite evidence that any specific preventative intervention will modify the course of the illness.

Within the heterogeneous group of conditions represented by the term *dementia*, the strongest case for intervention would appear to hold for vascular dementia. Vascular dementia itself is thought to involve a range of different processes, but modifying cardiovascular risk factors may delay the onset and reduce the severity of cerebrovascular disease, in turn reducing the risk of developing vascular dementia.

GPs may be questioned by their patients as to whether other strategies can prevent or delay the onset of dementia. These may include 'exercising the mind' (such as learning a second language or musical instrument or perhaps completing the daily crossword), supplements, diets and relaxation strategies, such as yoga and meditation. The best response would be to first ascertain that no harm will be caused by the activity, if indeed such an assessment is possible, and then to offer realistic but positive encouragement. Once again, however, there is no evidence of any of these strategies having a positive impact on the disease process.

The role of primary care in diagnosis and management

Current National Institute for Health and Care Excellence (NICE) guidance states that a diagnosis of dementia should be made by a specialist, but there may be times when it is better for this to be carried out in primary care. One reason would be patient choice, but other reasons would include the severity of the dementia and the mobility of the patient.

The assessment of a patient with cognitive impairment in primary care can take longer than the standard 10-minute general practice consultation. History taking can be time consuming. It is a process that may span several consultations, as supporting histories from family and carers are often required.

Before making an assessment, it is important to consider the issue of consent. Consultations regarding possible dementia are unusual

in that the patient is often brought by a relative or carer and may not be aware of the reason for the consultation. Consent for assessment must first be obtained if a patient has the capacity. If not, any further medical intervention must be in that person's best interests. This can make an already challenging consultation more difficult. Initial assessment is summarised in Box 10.2.

Box 10.2 **Initial assessment in primary care**

- History of the cognitive impairment – onset/pattern of deficits
- Symptoms of potential differential diagnoses, for example, depression/delirium
- Cardiovascular risk profile
- Consider screening for depression using, for example, PHQ9 score
- Physical examination
- Investigations to exclude differential diagnoses:
  - FBC full blood count
  - B12/folate
  - U&Es urea and electrolytes
  - TSH thyroid stimulating hormone
  - LFT liver function tests
  - Bone (calcium)
  - HBA1c
- Also consider:
  - MSU mid stream urine
  - CXR chest X-ray
  - Computed tomography (CT) or magnetic resonance imaging (MRI) head
- A test of cognitive function

Assessing cognitive function

Through the standard process of taking a history, it may become apparent that the patient has a degree of cognitive impairment. In order to establish the degree of impairment, a cognitive assessment tool may be used (Box 10.3).

Box 10.3 **Some examples of cognitive assessment scales used in the diagnosis of dementia in primary care**

- Abbreviated Mental Test Score (AMT)
- Mini Mental State Examination (MMSE)
- Modified Mini Mental State Examination (3MS)
- General Practitioner Assessment of Cognition (GPCOG) Scale
- Six-Item Cognitive Impairment Test (6CIT)

Ideally, a scale for use in primary care should be sensitive, specific, easy to use and fit into a standard 10-minute consultation. Unfortunately, none of the currently available scales completely fit all these criteria. A number of scales have been developed specifically for primary care, and it may be that one of these is the most appropriate to use, for example, the GPCOG.

It is important for a clinician to familiarise himself or herself with at least one scale and become proficient in its use. When using a scale, it may be necessary to take into account other factors that may affect a patient's performance (Box 10.4).

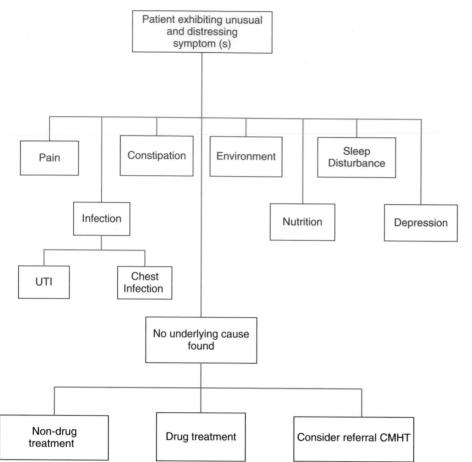

Figure 10.1 Suggested approach for the management of a patient presenting with behavioural and psychological symptoms of dementia (BPSD).

> **Box 10.4 Factors affecting performance when assessing patients using a cognitive assessment scale**
>
> - Educational level
> - Skills
> - Prior level of functioning and attainment
> - Language
> - Sensory impairment
> - Psychiatric illness
> - Physical or neurological problems

If significant cognitive impairment is identified, the following interventions should be considered:

- Medication review – minimise use of medications that adversely affect cognitive functioning.
- Ascertain whether the patient is still driving and whether a Class 1 or 2 licence is held. Advise accordingly.
- Identify nominated carer and establish if additional formal care is required.
- Introduce the concept of advance decision planning.
- Have a full discussion of the nature of the condition with the patient, relatives and carers.
- Referral to a secondary care service if required.

The team approach

All members of the primary health care team have a role to play in the care of patients with dementia. From the viewpoint of a patient with cognitive impairment, the entire process of accessing and receiving treatment or advice at a GP surgery can present difficulties. Telephoning to make an appointment, registering on arrival in the building (especially if 'self-check-in' machines are in use), finding the correct waiting room and answering the call of the clinician can all be problematic. It is therefore important to raise awareness of dementia and the potential problems facing patients in every member of the team.

Once a diagnosis has been made, the patient with dementia can benefit from contact and support from a variety of other individuals and organisations (Table 10.1). Provision of these services varies from area to area. Increasingly, these services are attached to primary care teams, facilitating improved teamwork and cooperation.

Patient-centred care

The main focus of the primary care team should be to enable the patient to exploit the full potential of the abilities that he or she still possesses. This is frequently referred to as 'living well with dementia'. A well-established approach to this is the concept of patient-centred care (Box 10.5). This approach is increasingly being adopted in care homes with excellent results.

> Box 10.5 **Patient-centred care**
>
> Caring for a patient with dementia should take account of the following aspects.
>
> - The human value of people with dementia, regardless of age or cognitive impairment, and those who care for them
> - The individuality of people with dementia, with their unique personality and life experiences among the influences on their response to the dementia
> - The importance of the perspective of the person with dementia
> - The importance of relationships and interactions with others to the person with dementia, and their potential for promoting well-being

Advance decision planning

A vital role of the primary care team is to introduce the concept of advance decision planning to the patient with dementia, his or her family and carers. Important issues regarding the future medical management of the patient can be addressed while the patient still has the capacity to make decisions. Without this process, the patient may be subjected to unnecessary and unwanted interventions later in the disease process, when the patient no longer has the capacity to make decisions.

Table 10.1 Sources of support for patients with dementia.

Dementia advisors	They provide support for patients, family and carers throughout the course of the illness.
Admiral Nurses	Specialist mental health nurses with a particular interest and additional training in dementia. Provide specialist support to the primary care team.
Community mental health team	Multidisciplinary team that may include psychiatrists, community mental health nurses and occupational therapists. Provide specialist support to the primary care team.
Third-sector organisations, for example: • Alzheimer's Society • Age UK • MIND • Local carer organisations	Provide information, advice and support for all aspects of dementia care. A wide range of local services are provided.

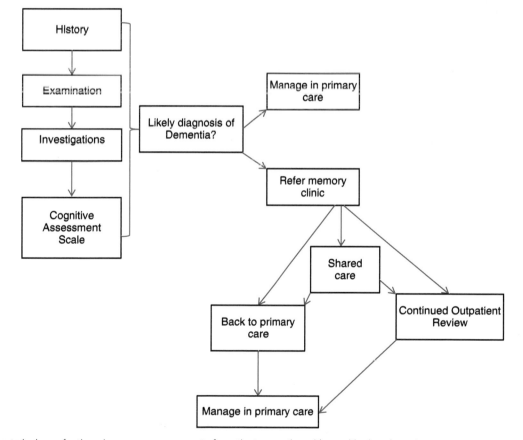

Figure 10.2 Suggested scheme for the primary care management of a patient presenting with cognitive impairment.

Dementia in care homes

A high percentage of patients with dementia on a GP list are likely to be living in a care home. It is estimated that 80% of care-home residents have some form of dementia. More severe cases may need care in a nursing home specialising in the care of patients with dementia (Elderly Mentally Ill EMI Home). The primary care team is responsible for organising regular reviews of these patients, focusing on both the physical and psychological aspects of their care. Partnership working between primary care and care-home staff is an essential component of good management in this area.

In addition, a GP may be asked to review a patient exhibiting behaviour unusual for that individual, often referred to as the behavioural and psychological symptoms of dementia (BPSD). The patient is often unable to give a coherent history. Efforts should be made to establish and treat the cause of the patient's distress (Figure 10.1). If no cause can be established, non-pharmacological approaches should first be considered. The use of antipsychotic medication should be reserved as a last resort, and then used only for a short period, pending a review of the management strategy. Referral to the local community mental health team may be required if these measures are not successful.

The future of dementia management in primary care

In the early stages of the condition, the current role of the GP is to identify patients with a possible dementia and plan their future management accordingly. It may be possible for the GP to make a diagnosis of dementia, particularly if the patient is severely affected. Currently, a diagnosis will usually be confirmed following a referral to secondary care.

Shared care arrangements may be in place between primary and secondary care for the initial stages of management. Once the patient has been assessed, started on treatment where appropriate and stabilised on treatment, the patient will be discharged back to primary care (Figure 10.2).

Looking to the future, perhaps the main issue for primary care is to establish to what extent patients with dementia should be managed in the primary care setting. For example, is it appropriate or desirable for a GP to make a diagnosis of dementia, initiate treatment and monitor the course of the illness without referral to secondary care? Clearly, non-clinical factors will play an important role in determining the answer to this question, and commissioners will need to make increasingly important decisions around the distribution of resources in this area.

In the future, all sectors will need to work together in a dynamic and forward thinking way, as failing to address and effectively manage this group of patients will have major clinical and resource implications.

Further reading

Alzheimer's Society. *Mapping the Dementia Gap* 2012 alzheimers.org.uk.

Bechtel C. If you build it, will they come? Designing truly patient-centered health care. Health Affairs 2010; **29**(5):914–920.

General Practitioner Assessment of Cognition (GPCOG) found on www.gpcog.com.au

Institute on Medicine. *Crossing the Quality Chasm: A New Health System for the 21st Century*. National Academies Press: Washington, DC, 2001.

Wilson JMG, Jungner G. Principles and practice of screening for disease. WHO Chronicle 1968; **22**(11):473.

CHAPTER 11

Dementia in the Acute Hospital

Elizabeth Ward[1], Daryl L. Leung[2], and Georgios Theodoulou[3]

[1] Royal Wolverhampton NHS Trust, Wolverhampton, UK
[2] Elderly Care and Dementia Service Royal Wolverhampton NHS Trust, Wolverhampton, UK
[3] Worcestershire Health and Care NHS Trust, Worcestershire, UK

OVERVIEW

- At least a quarter of people in hospital have dementia. Fifty percent of people with dementia are undiagnosed.

- People with dementia stay longer in hospital compared with someone without dementia, and are less likely to be discharged home.

- A hospital admission for a person with dementia can be challenging to them, their carer/relatives and the hospital.

- Better dementia care in hospitals is everyone's responsibility. It has been shown to improve outcome and save money.

- Admission prevention, dementia-friendly hospitals and mental health liaison are three ways to improve dementia care in the acute setting.

Introduction

At any time, a quarter of people in hospital will have dementia, and for over half of these patients, dementia will not have been diagnosed. The demographic change that is occurring in the community is reflected in the admissions to hospital. According to the Dementia Action Alliance 2013, there are currently 800,000 people living with dementia in the UK, and this number is expected to rise to over one million by 2025. The current financial cost of dementia to the UK is over £23 billion a year.

This chapter deals with the experiences of people with dementia in hospital, the challenges they and the hospital services may face, and how this very important area of health care can and must be improved.

Challenges to the person with dementia

Coming into hospital can be a bewildering and distressing time for anyone. These feelings become more intense for a person with impaired ability to remember, understand or communicate. The first 48 hours of an admission may involve several changes of location – from A+E, to an assessment unit to a ward, as well as trips to other departments for tests.

ABC of Dementia, First Edition. Edited by Bernard Coope and Felicity Richards.
© 2014 John Wiley & Sons, Ltd. Published 2014 by John Wiley & Sons, Ltd.

The strict structure of the day with meal times, medication rounds and ward rounds regiment the time, and the environment is unfamiliar, noisy and crowded. It is not surprising that, as a result, a person with dementia may call out for help, ask repeated questions or set off to explore the ward hoping to find their way home. The absence of familiar relatives will add to this searching and need for attachment.

Such behaviour may be seen as 'difficult' on a ward, especially if irritation shows itself with angry words or actions. Sedating medication frequently follows, significantly increasing the risk of a fall or chest infection, and further reducing a person's ability to communicate their needs. Even the simple process of ensuring adequate nutrition and hydration can become challenging, and weight loss is common.

Hospitals are frightening, upsetting and dangerous places for people with dementia. It is hard to keep dignity and there is a very high chance of dying in hospital or never returning home.

Challenges to family

Most people living with dementia in the community rely on a carer to support them and this is usually a member of the immediate family. As a person's dementia progresses, the carer will spend more time in the company of their relative, providing comfort and support, helping with shopping and other household tasks and also often providing high levels of personal care. This can be a stressful experience but it also leads to a strong bond.

When a person with dementia enters hospital and becomes a patient, he or she enters a world of confidentiality. Hospital staff trained in the need to maintain confidentiality can be reluctant to discuss health matters with a relative. The relative can feel like an unwelcome spectator, confined to visiting times with little engagement around the planning and provision of care within the hospital. Their wisdom of caring for their family member is lost to the hospital. The personal likes and dislikes, the tell-tale signs of pain that a close member of the family will know or the fact that the person won't admit to not hearing well are missed – facts that would help hospital staff provide good care. Previously expressed wishes about care that may be very familiar and could guide important decision-making are unknown to those wishing to help the patient.

Challenges to the hospital

Hospitals are increasingly the setting of rapid and high-tech assessment and treatment. From gathering a history to gaining consent, to carrying out physical examinations or invasive investigations, the cooperation of patients is essential to help this process work efficiently.

What then of the person who can't say what is the matter? Are they in pain? How long have they been short of breath for? What about consent or involvement in planning? And how to respond to the man who walks around the ward messing with another patient's drip, or asking how he will get home to his mother despite being over eighty? When nursing staff are carrying out skilled procedures, who will ensure the patients have eaten their meal?

When the process of investigation and treatment has run its course and it is time for discharge, this can be a much more complex process for a person with dementia and lengths of stay are significantly longer. The person with dementia then starts to be referred to as a 'bed blocker'.

How do hospitals make themselves unfriendly? See Table 11.1.

Better dementia care in hospital

There are three parallel approaches to helping the experiences of people with dementia who need hospital care.

1 Admission prevention
2 Dementia-friendly hospitals
3 Mental health liaison

Admission prevention

If it is so problematic to be in hospital with dementia, then the obvious first point to address is whether the admission was needed in the first place or whether there are alternative ways of providing treatment. Strategies include the following:

Careful management of chronic conditions to prevent acute episodes;
'Virtual ward' services in the community to provide intensive and specialised care out of hospital;
Better social care to avoid carer breakdown and emergency calls;
Inreach into care homes – specialist teams addressing physical or mental health needs for those in care homes to prevent admission;
Better advanced planning and palliative care.

Table 11.1 How do hospitals make themselves dementia unfriendly?

Multiple ward moves
Structured timetable for the day
Sending patients alone to X-ray/clinics
Lack of awareness/identification of dementia
Lack of appreciation of pain
Sedation and use of anti-psychotics
Closed visiting times for carers and relatives

Admission avoidance can be a better way of providing care. However, a word of ethical caution is needed. 'Helping people with dementia stay out of hospital' is very different from 'keeping people with dementia out of hospital'. Those with dementia deserve good care like anyone else.

The dementia-friendly hospital

With a lot of imagination and hard work it is possible to change the way a hospital stay is experienced by a person with dementia. Hospitals are beginning to recognise the unaddressed needs of patients with dementia in the acute hospital setting. In order to understand how this can be achieved, the following example in Box 11.1 a 'dementia-friendly hospital' will be explored.

Box 11.1 **A dementia-friendly hospital**

At New Cross Hospital in Wolverhampton, UK, a package of changes have been introduced to demonstrate a holistic approach to dementia care at all levels in the Trust, enshrined by a culture of fostering best care for patients with dementia. The prevalence of dementia in the acute hospital is about 40%, of which only half have a diagnosis pre-admission. Therefore, a great need arises for an integrated service to deliver the best care to patients. The Dementia Care Bundle addresses these needs by using the following three approaches:

Person-centred care with involvement of carers and relatives
An environmental understanding of both physical and emotional needs
Hydration and nutrition.

Integral to this is the 'About Me' document, which is designed to give the reader a greater understanding of the patient and to devise an individual care plan tailored to the needs of that person. All aspects of care are considered including preferences of food and drink, behaviours that may indicate a need to go to the toilet or other signs of distress and how to de-escalate them.

Person-centred care with involvement of carers and relatives

Involves communication with patients, relatives and carers in a manner that is compassionate and personalised. The 'About Me' document highlights a person's preferences, topics of interests, types of behaviour to be identified and how to recognise signs of distress.

The environment

Calm and friendly emotional environment with clear orientation and signage and more open access to visiting carers and relatives. De-clutter the environment and encourage mobility.

Hydration and nutrition

A separate area for eating, ensuring adequate intake of fluid and food that the patient prefers is identified in the 'About Me' document; volunteers and relatives also support meal times.

The role of relatives and carers

Relatives and carers of patients with dementia in hospital are a grossly under-used resource. They can provide invaluable information about their relative for care planning. Knowledge of the person's likes and dislikes, behaviour (changes in mood/distress/pain), wishes and opinions can help shape care, and can be used in order to facilitate shared care decision-making in the person's best interests. These discussions can also highlight the relative's expectations of medical care, plan end-of-life care, resuscitation decisions and preferences for place of death. In the case of Wolverhampton, this information is used in the 'About Me' document.

Engaging with families requires a change in culture in hospital staff. Hospital professionals learn early in their training about the importance of confidentiality and have the misguided belief that the law prohibits them discussing a patient's care with members of the family. This is not the case for those who lack decision-making capacity. In fact, the Code of Practice for the Mental Capacity Act 2005 strongly encourages discussions with family on key aspects of care and treatment.

It is important that carer burden is acknowledged; around two thirds of people with dementia are cared for in the community and by unpaid carers. Depression in carers can lead to a reduction in quality of life and increased unplanned admissions to secondary care. Setting up hospital care groups can help alleviate their stress, provide support and an environment to improve the hospital experience of all (Table 11.2).

Table 11.2 Other ways of making a hospital 'dementia friendly'.

Prioritisation of patients with dementia for least number of ward moves and timely investigations. To move within hours, if needed preferably with relative or carer escort.

Flexibility in mealtimes, washing and waking. Patients with dementia don't necessarily fit in the routine of the hospital; relatives and carers to support the above-mentioned aspects.

Escort service to X-ray/outpatient (OP) clinics by member of staff, relative or volunteers. Dementia champions in all areas of the organisation such as porters, outpatients, ambulance service, radiology, orthopaedics and elderly care.

Education for staff regarding dementia, and the importance of recognising those undiagnosed.

Staff recognition of pain (using advice of carers/relatives) – patients with dementia commonly receive only one-third of the analgesia for neck of femur fractures compared to patients without dementia on the same ward.

Avoid oversedation: The alternative to sedation for most circumstances requires anticipation by staff of situations that may cause distress and reducing these. If the only option is anti-psychotics, short-term use is recommended and there *must* be a plan for tapered reduction.

Greater open access to relatives and carers to help in care of the patient with dementia. Start support groups for relatives and carers, open up communication, improve quality-of-care experience and support for discharge planning

Table 11.3 Outlining the role of Mental Health Liaison Services for older adults.

Provide timely assessment, diagnosis and treatment of mental health needs for any older person who is currently in a general hospital

Facilitate better communication between patient, carers and treating clinicians

Teaching and training of acute hospital staff on the 4 D's – dementia, delirium, depression and dignity

Provide a link to community mental services, Admiral Nurses and voluntary dementia support services

Joint ward rounds and mutlidisciplinary team (MDT) meetings with social workers, Occupational Therapist (OT), nurses, geriatricians

Contribute to Trust governance activities and structures, for example, audit, complaints, safeguarding committees, dementia steering groups

Mental health liaison

Mental Health Liaison Services are provided by specialist mental health practitioners working in an acute hospital setting and deliver assessment, management and treatment for a wide variety of mental health issues. Although hospital liaison was specifically developed for adults of working age, these services have been recognised as an important aspect of inpatient care for people with dementia. It has been demonstrated that having mental health services based in general hospitals for older people leads to reduced length of stay, reduced readmission rates and reduced institutionalisation rates.

It is not uncommon for a person with dementia to complete an episode of care in an acute hospital with no reference to their cognitive impairment. Moreover, given that a hospital inpatient stay requires patients to make potentially very serious healthcare decisions, the legal framework (Mental Capacity Act 2005) for decision-making was and still is largely not understood or applied by non-mental health specialist staff in acute hospitals. With more widespread older peoples' mental health services, the quality of care for people with dementia (and delirium) is changing.

The influence of a specialist mental health team in a hospital has a very powerful effect on staff practices – from modelling of interactions through to dissemination of knowledge and best practice guidance, even if not all patients with dementia are seen directly (Table 11.3).

Delirium in the acute hospital setting

Delirium is a major cause of morbidity and mortality in patients in hospital, especially in older people and those who already have dementia. Delirium can last from a few days up to 2–3 months. Chronic delirium is a major cause of death, increased hospital stay, prescription of antipsychotic drugs and increased likelihood of being discharged into placement. Delirium is a complex neuropsychiatric syndrome characterised by

- an acute onset
- fluctuating course
- perceptual abnormalities: visual or auditory hallucinations

- global cognitive impairment: difficulty focusing attention /disorganised thinking
- altered level of consciousness (don't be fooled by lucid intervals; this is characteristic of delirium).

Two main types arise:

1. Hypoactive – quiet, lethargic, marked increased mortality because of delayed recognition in symptoms by health care professionals.
2. Hyperactive delirium – hyperaroused, irritable, lability of mood. Perceptual abnormalities are prominent. Patients with hyperactive delirium are more likely to be prescribed sedatives and anti-psychotics (Box 11.2).

Box 11.2 **Types of semi-purposeful repetitive movements may indicate delirium, first described by Hippocrates**

Carphology: the plucking or picking at bedclothes and clothing
Floccillation: plucking in the air

The causes of delirium are often multifactorial, and treatment should be tailored towards identifying potential causes and treating these accordingly. Sedation should be kept to a minimum. Educating staff about preventing delirium, and diagnosing it early (especially hypoactive delirium) will greatly reduce mortality, morbidity and length of hospital stay.

Conclusion

A large number of patients in acute hospitals have dementia, and over half of these individuals are undiagnosed. The number of people with dementia is increasing rapidly, and the NHS must look at ways of improving services to provide more appropriate care at home, reduce inappropriate/unnecessary admissions and ensure that if a person with dementia has to access the acute setting, their experience is timely, effective and dementia friendly. Education for staff on early identification of dementia, the needs of people with dementia and the importance of family/carer involvement is crucial in order to manage all aspects of care in a person's best interests with their wishes in mind (Box 11.3).

Box 11.3 **Case examples**

An 83-year-old man with vascular dementia had acute delirium. He remained mobile, was at risk of falls and was being managed on a 'winter pressures' ward. Over the weekend, he was moved twice before finally coming to the dementia ward. He was sedated because of 'agitation'. During these moves, he became bedbound and nursing records documented complaints of right leg pain. His family were understandably concerned about his reduced mobility and continued to complain of pain on mobilising during physio. An X-ray of the right hip revealed a fractured neck of femur.

Lessons learnt

Agitation should be taken seriously, and a cause found.

Listen to members of the MDT, this man could have had his fracture diagnosed sooner as his nursing notes indicated pain in the right hip 2–3 days before he was mobilised by physiotherapists.

Pain can be very difficult to assess in patients with dementia, and generally patients with dementia are given far less pain relief than those without dementia.

Case two

An 87-year-old lady with end-stage dementia is bedbound. Her devoted daughter is her main carer. Her general practitioner (GP) had given oral antibiotics for a chest infection 2 weeks previously. She is now much more unwell but without venous access. Her daughter has been feeding her nutritional drinks on a pink mouthwash sponge; and 200 ml takes 90 min. The nurses are unhappy as this is too time consuming for them but do not invite the daughter to do this instead.

Lessons learnt

In this situation, encouraging the daughter to feed her mother should have been a priority.

Nasogastric tubes can be appropriate in certain situations and certainly for the short-term; however, this must be discussed with relatives, and have a clear purpose and a clear plan.

This case also highlights the importance of end-of-life discussions and prognosis, including ceiling of care, how to treat further infections and preference for place of death. This not only manages expectations but also allows relatives to plan for the future.

Further reading

Dementia Action Alliance www.dementiaaction.org.uk

CHAPTER 12

Dementia and the Law

Felicity A. Richards[1] and Jelena Jankovic[2]

[1]Worcestershire Health and Care NHS Trust, Worcestershire, UK
[2]Dudley and Walsall Mental Health Partnership Trust, Dudley, UK

OVERVIEW

- A diagnosis of dementia does not automatically equate to a lack of decision-making capacity.
- The Mental Capacity Act 2005 (MCA) underpins many aspects of the management of incapacitous persons – both for physical and mental health decisions.
- The assessment of a person's capacity must be based on the ability to make a specific decision at the time it needs to be made, not the ability to make decisions in general.
- The capacity assessment for specific decisions should be completed by the professional best suited to make that assessment – the 'decision-maker'. Indeed, the GMC – General Medical Council expects all doctors to be able to assess capacity in relation to their work.
- Advance care planning helps preserve autonomy and self-determination and should be encouraged in the early stages of dementia.

Introduction

A major concern for those developing dementia is the fear of losing control over their lives once they have lost the capacity to make decisions. A diagnosis of dementia does not automatically mean that a person lacks decision-making capacity. Patients are now diagnosed earlier at a time when they can plan care, nominate proxy decision-makers and hold on to their autonomy and self-determination. Future planning can also benefit those who will need to make decisions on behalf of an individual.

Health professionals are involved not only in encouraging and guiding people with dementia to plan for their future but also in assessing decision-making capacity and being part of proxy decision-making. The GMC expects all doctors to be able to assess a person's capacity in relation to their work. Decisions in dementia often involve balancing potential or actual risks with a person's autonomy, and should always be made in the best interests of that person.

This chapter covers legislation regarding the Mental Capacity Act, Mental Health Act and Deprivation of Liberty Safeguards (DoLS), as

well as covering advance planning and some common ethical dilemmas faced in dementia.

Legislation

1 Mental Capacity Act 2005 (MCA 2005)
2 Mental Health Act 1983 (MHA 2007)
3 Deprivation of Liberty Safeguards (DoLS)

Mental Capacity Act 2005

Mental capacity is simply the ability to make a decision. The Mental Capacity Act 2005, which applies to England and Wales, and the Adults with Incapacity (Scotland) Act 2000 offer a legal framework for assessing capacity, and making decisions on behalf of those who lack mental capacity to make decisions for themselves. The statutory principles of the MCA 2005, as outlined in Box 12.1, are there to protect people who lack capacity, and to help them where possible, take part in decisions that affect them (Box 12.1).

Box 12.1 **Five statutory principles of the MCA 2005**

1 A presumption of capacity, unless established that an individual lacks capacity
2 All practicable steps taken to help an individual make a decision
3 Individuals are entitled to make unwise decisions
4 An act done/decision made on behalf of an individual who lacks capacity must be done/made in their best interests
5 The least restrictive option should be explored

Assessing mental capacity

It is a requirement that every health professional should be able to assess an individual's capacity. Capacity is assessed via the two-stage test of capacity, followed by an assessment of an individual's ability to make a specific decision, as outlined in Box 12.2.

Under the Mental Capacity Act, a person is deemed to lack capacity, if

- there is an impairment or disturbance (e.g. a disability, condition or trauma) that affects the way the mind or brain works, and
- the impairment or disturbance means that the person is unable to make a specific decision at the time it needs to be made.

ABC of Dementia, First Edition. Edited by Bernard Coope and Felicity Richards.
© 2014 John Wiley & Sons, Ltd. Published 2014 by John Wiley & Sons, Ltd.

Box 12.2 **Two-stage test of capacity**

1 Does the person have an impairment of the mind or brain, or is there some sort of disturbance affecting the way the mind or brain works (temporary or permanent)?

2 If so, does that impairment or disturbance mean that the person is unable to make the decision in question at the time it needs to be made?

Assessing the ability to make a specific decision

- Does the person have a general understanding of what decision needs to be made and the need to make it?
- Does the person have a general understanding of the likely consequences of making, or not making, this decision?
- Is the person able to understand, retain, use and weigh up the information relevant to this decision?
- Can the person communicate the decision?

Important points

- The assessment of an individual's capacity must be based on the ability to make a specific decision at the time it needs to be made, not the ability to make decisions in general.
- The capacity assessment for specific decisions should be completed by the professional best suited to make that assessment – the 'decision-maker', that is, an ambulance crew conveying an individual to hospital, a social worker assessing placement decisions or a doctor deciding on treatment.
- If the decision is more complex, involvement of other health professionals may be necessary.

Relationship between the Mental Health Act and Mental Capacity Act

In very rare circumstances, professionals may need to think about using the Mental Health Act 2007 to detain and treat somebody with dementia who lacks capacity to consent to treatment, rather than using the MCA 2005.

A situation where this need may arise is if an individual is severely disturbed, and needs to be admitted to hospital for their own health and/or safety, or the safety of others with the intention to treat a mental disorder. It must be stressed however, that dementia care services, wherever possible, should be community based. Inpatient admissions increase the risk of morbidity, mortality and institutionalization for those with dementia. These decisions are often complex, and guidance for determining which framework to use is constantly evolving in the context of a growing number of case law decisions. Involvement of secondary mental health services may be necessary.

Deprivation of Liberty Safeguards (DoLS)

DoLS provides an independent assessment process for individuals who lack capacity and, as a consequence, may need to be deprived of their liberty in order for care to be provided in a safe environment (in their best interests).

The MCA 2005 led to the introduction of DoLS, which became law on April 1, 2009.

Common situations where DoLS are used include care-home settings and hospital wards. If an individual who lacks capacity is at risk of being deprived of their liberty, or is deprived of their liberty, the Care-Home Manager or Hospital Ward Manager, are obliged to apply to their supervisory body (Local Health Board/Authority) for an authorisation of deprivation of liberty. For example, a gentleman with advanced dementia who continuously attempts to leave his Care Home needs restrictions placed on his freedom (a locked door policy), to keep him safe. In deciding on the need for a DoLS assessment, health care professionals are not involved, other than in the context of an advisory role if necessary.

Making decisions for the future: advance care planning

Earlier diagnosis offers many people with dementia the opportunity to be able to plan more effectively for a time when their capacity to make decisions may be affected. These decisions may revolve around health matters and financial decision (see Box 12.3).

Box 12.3 **Advance care planning and nomination of proxy-decision makers**

Health decisions: advance care planning and nomination of a proxy decision-maker(s) in advance of losing capacity:

1 Advance Statements
2 Advance Decisions to Refuse Treatment
3 Lasting Power of Attorney (LPA) for personal welfare and health

Financial decisions: nomination of a proxy decision-maker(s) in advance of losing capacity

1 LPA for property and finances
2 Enduring Power of Attorney before October 2007. Replaced by LPA.

Care planning: for those who lack decision-making capacity and have not nominated a proxy decision-maker(s) for health and welfare, and property and finances

1 Court of Protection application
2 Allocation of an Independent Mental Capacity Advocate (IMCA)

Health decisions
Advance Statements

Advance Statements are a crucial aspect of advance care planning. An 'advance statement' is a broad term used to describe a range of wishes for future treatment, including treatment preferences and refusals, preferences on important aspects of home life/personal life and appointment of a surrogate decision-maker (see Box 12.4).

Advance decision to refuse treatment (ADRT)

ADRTs are usually incorporated into the wider advance statement of a person with dementia. ADRTs are legally binding if made at a time when a person has the mental capacity to make such a decision

Box 12.4 **Advance Statements: what they can include**

Instructions about medical treatment

Medication preferences and refusals (and reasons why) including refusal/preferences for ECT. Advance Decisions to Refuse Treatment (ADRT) often included in advance statement
Preferred method of de-escalating crisis
Description of response to hospital admissions
Preference of hospital/hospital alternatives
Appointment of surrogate decisions maker/LPA

Instructions about personal care

Individuals to be notified of hospital admission, about care of finances, dependants or pets
People not authorised to visit during hospitalisation
Dietary preferences
Assisted devices (e.g. dentures)

and the decision is applicable to the given situation. For refusal of life-sustaining treatment, an ADRT must be in writing, signed and witnessed with a clear statement that it is applicable even if life is at risk.

Lasting Power of Attorney for personal welfare and health

Individuals who have the capacity can complete a LPA to appoint an attorney(s) to make proxy decisions on their behalf at a time when they have lost capacity. An LPA can be taken out for both (i) property and finances and (ii) personal welfare and health.

Personal welfare can include the power for an attorney to consent to or refuse medical treatment on an individual's behalf if this is expressed in the LPA. An LPA giving an attorney a decision to refuse treatment will invalidate any previous advance decision to refuse treatment made by the individual. An attorney cannot consent to or refuse treatment for a mental disorder for a patient detained under MHA 1983.

LPAs can only be used once registered with the Office of the Public Guardian. Attorneys must always act in a person's best interests and take note of a person's prior wishes/choices where applicable. End-of-life decisions can be incorporated into both Advance Statements and LPAs, as described in Chapter 13.

Financial decisions

Enduring Power of Attorney and Lasting Power of Attorney for property and finances

Enduring Power of Attorney (EPA) were replaced in October 2007 by LPA for property and finances. An EPA is still valid, whether it has been registered at the Court of Protection or not, provided that both the donor of the power and the attorney/s signed the document before October 1, 2007. An EPA can be used while a person still has mental capacity for financial decisions only, provided an individual can consent to its use. Once an individual is felt to lack capacity regarding finances, the EPA must be registered with the Office of the Public Guardian. The attorney/s can use finances for essential

purposes (food/bills) whilst the EPA registration is being processed, no larger financial transactions can take place.

Court of Protection/Deputyship

For those individuals who lack capacity to appoint a proxy decision-maker(s), a deputy can apply to the Court of Protection (CoP). The court can decide whether a person has capacity to make a particular decision for himself or herself, and can appoint deputies. If there is no one who can be a deputy, the CoP has the power to make decisions on behalf of an individual.

Both attorneys (LPA) and deputies (CoP) have to act in that person's best interests, and expenditure is accountable to the CoP. Failure to do so could amount to abuse, physical or financial or both, and the CoP can remove deputies or attorneys who fail to carry out their duties.

Difficulties around capacity

There will be times when it is not clear if a person with dementia has the capacity to make a particular decision. If felt to have capacity, that person will be free to make a choice, even if it appears unwise or indeed risky. However, if deemed to lack capacity, someone else will make a decision for them. Although made in the person's best interests, the proxy decision may go against an individual's previous wishes.

Decisions in dementia, therefore, frequently involve balancing risks with a person's autonomy. Professionals and carers often and understandably strive to minimise or alleviate as much risk as possible, but can fail to recognise that forgoing activities that promote independence (just in case potential risks could ensue), could result in an individual missing out on the benefits.

Treating an incapacitous person

Treating an incapacitous person in his or her own best interest is the underlying purpose of MCA 2005. This requires health care professionals to determine a patient's personal beliefs, values and wishes that are likely to influence important treatment decisions. Engagement with families/carers/advocates when making a decision is of great importance and can shape shared-care decisions. Discussions with these parties are highlighted in the MCA 2005. Examining Advance Statements, including ADRT, and identifying attorneys/deputies is part of this process. Box 12.5 outlines the steps to be taken in treating a person who lacks capacity.

Box 12.5 **Steps to be taken in treating an incapacitious patient**

1 Exploring person's wishes about treatment (including Advance Statements and Advance Decisions to Refuse Treatment).
2 Identifying those who have a surrogate decision-maker (LPA for personal welfare/health or COP).
3 Providing independent help to an incapacitous person to make decisions (appointing an IMCA); see subsequent text.
4 Formulating a treatment plan based on best interest decisions (including covert medication prescribing); see subsequent text.

Independent Mental Capacity Advocate (IMCA) service

If an individual who lacks capacity has no one else to support them an IMCA will be instructed to support and represent that individual in decision-making, providing an independent safeguard. Decisions include treatment of serious medical conditions, placement/accommodation issues, care reviews and adult protection cases. IMCAs can have access to health and social care records. When reaching a conclusion on a proposed decision in a person's best interests, the information gained by an IMCA must be taken into account.

Covert medication prescribing

Under the provisions of the MCA 2005, if a patient with dementia lacks the decision-making capacity for treatment, and medication is felt necessary to save a person's life or prevent deterioration in their health, covert medication can be given if:

1 it is agreed that it is in the person's best interests to do so;
2 no advance statement including ADRTs apply;
3 this is the only method of ensuring that medication is taken.

It is the prescriber's responsibility to assess capacity. It should be documented clearly as a 'Best Interests' decision in a person's care plan, with full involvement of family/carers/proxy decision-makers, and other health professionals involved in care (doctors, pharmacists). The administration should be in the least restrictive form of all options available. Documentation should be medication specific and the administration method used should not affect drug efficacy.

Dementia, driving and the law

A diagnosis of dementia does not automatically exclude an individual from driving; however, as dementia progresses, the ability to drive safely will eventually be lost. Once a diagnosis of dementia has been shared with an individual, the doctor's role is to inform that person of their legal obligation to notify the DVLA and insurance company of their diagnosis. Not doing so may invalidate their insurance policy, and result in a £1000 fine from the DVLA. The DVLA will then ask for a practical report, either from the person's general practitioner (GP) or psychiatrist, confirming the diagnosis and asking brief questions about medications, and the impact their dementia has on decision-making and judgement. An annual review will usually take place. This process relies on self-reporting, but if there are serious concerns about an individual's safety, a medical professional can break confidentiality and inform the DVLA in writing.

Importantly, cognitive assessment on its own does not determine if an individual is safe to drive. If there is uncertainty, an in-car driving assessment should be considered.

Rates of crashes in drivers with dementia are low for up to three years after disease onset. The consequences of revoking a licence are far reaching and include increasing isolation from friends and family (especially rural living), difficulties in accessing shops/day centres and is an independent factor for entry into a nursing home; Breen, 2007. BMJ.

Conclusion

An early diagnosis of dementia allows people to plan for their future. This enables individuals to feel that their wishes and opinions will be taken seriously at a time when others may have to make decisions on their behalf. Decisions in more advanced dementia often require balancing a person's autonomy with potential risks. A person's best interests should be at the heart of all decisions.

Scenarios

1. Alice, an 84-year-old lady with a diagnosis of moderate Alzheimer's disease, falls and fractures her hip. Without appropriate treatment in hospital, Alice may die. Alice refuses to come into hospital, hitting out at paramedics, who then refuse to transport her in the ambulance as she is not 'consenting'. She has not got a nominated proxy decision-maker, or an advance statement.

Issues

*Capacity assessment. Alice lacks decision-making capacity regarding her life-threatening injury and need for treatment. All health care professionals are expected to be able to assess an individual's capacity. The decision-maker regarding her transport from home to hospital to receive treatment is the paramedic. It is in Alice's best interests to be taken to hospital to prevent further deterioration or death. If Alice is left at home and not treated, this could be viewed as neglect, and potentially carry a custodial sentence. Importantly, the MCA would offer protection against this decision, and would support the paramedic in transporting Alice to hospital, even with a temporary restriction of her liberty.

2. Bill, a 76-year-old with mild vascular dementia, lives alone. He is self-neglecting at times, losing weight and there are issues around medication compliance. He is on six different medications, which he receives monthly in individual boxes. He has been found on the floor following falls twice in the past 3 months. He is felt to have capacity to make decisions regarding his social situation, and would accept more care. His wish is to remain at home with his dog. His son and daughter phone Bill's GP urgently requesting for Bill to be moved into a residential home as they are his attorneys under LPA for personal welfare and health.

Issues

*Capacity assessment for staying at home *and* capacity to consent to share information about his medical state. Bill still has capacity to decide on where he wishes to live and what information about his medical health/situation is shared with his family. Health professionals need to respect a capacitious person's wishes. In this case, the family need to be informed under the MCA 2005 that Bill is still able to make seemingly unwise/potentially risky decisions.

*Interventions that would allow Bill to live at home, and reduce potential risks could be explored further including a medication review with a Nomad system for his tablets, a care package, occupational therapist for home risk assessment and referral to a falls clinic.

*Even if the family has an LPA, Bill still has the capacity to decide on the above-mentioned aspects without the need for proxy decision-makers, and thus his decisions override his family's concerns.

Scenarios

3. A GP receives a phone call from a local care home stating that a person with dementia has 'gone mad' and needs to be moved immediately. The change in behaviour has been rapid, with the individual lashing out, responding to unseen stimuli and not sleeping.

Issues

* Rapid change in mental state points to a delirium that requires urgent medical assessment and treatment.

   * Decisions regarding the best place for treatment. Two options are (i) in the care home, (ii) hospital ward, not a psychiatric assessment ward. Often, familiar environments are best, and the least restrictive option. Care homes have a responsibility to increase staff if this is required, and cannot give notice of less than 28 days.

   * In these situations, one will use the MCA – it is in the person's best interests to treat, even if covert medication is required.

4. Betty, a 64-year-old lady diagnosed with a frontotemporal dementia (behavioural variant), begins to make increasingly unwise decisions, both financial and personal. Her son asks her to sign over properties into his name. Her GP feels that Betty lacks decision-making capacity around financial decisions and property.

Her son then requests you to sign the Court of Protection (COP3) form to appoint him as deputy. What do you do?

Issues

* Financial abuse. If there are any concerns about abuse of any form, vulnerable adult proceedings must be initiated. This amounts to probable financial abuse of a vulnerable adult, and the son could be prosecuted.

   * With regard to completing LPA or COP applications, one must be as certain as possible that the appointed deputy/attorney will act in that person's best interests. Health professionals can refuse to sign an LPA/COP3 form. The Office of the Public Guardian can be informed in writing of any concerns.

Further reading

Breen, DA et al. Driving and Dementia. *BMJ* 2007;**334**:1365.

Mental Capacity Act 2005 Code of Practice. www.justice.gov.uk/protecting-the-vulnerable/mental-capacity-act

Mental Health Act 2007 Code of Practice. www.nmhdu.org.uk/silo/files/mental-health-act-2007--new-roles.pdf

CHAPTER 13

End-of-Life Care in Dementia

Kay de Vries

Graduate School of Nursing, Midwifery & Health (GSNMH), Victoria University of Wellington, NZ
Association for Dementia Studies, University of Worcester, UK
University of Washington, Seattle, USA

OVERVIEW

- Understanding bereavement issues that arise for people with advanced dementia and their families is essential.
- Advance care planning for dementia should be initiated at an early assessment stage.
- Risk factors for mortality for people with dementia are not easily distinguished.
- The terminal stage for dementia is difficult to predict.
- People with dementia have symptoms and health care needs comparable with those with cancer at the end of life.
- Pain is under-reported and under-treated for people with dementia.

Introduction

Dementia is often an insidiously progressive illness that may advance over years. In many cases, families and professionals do not view dementia as a terminal illness and have little knowledge or understanding of the possible causes of death and what to expect as the illness progresses. However, people with dementia who are dying have significant health care needs and there are particular challenges and ethical dilemmas that both families and caregivers encounter.

A palliative care approach is proposed to be of benefit to people with dementia because of its emphasis on supportive care (including support for family). This approach encompasses: quality of life, symptom management, attention to formulating goals of care that guide medical decision-making, creation of a comfortable end-of-life experience and bereavement services.

Life-extending treatments are usually not appropriate. Discussions with the caregivers are central when evaluating an individual's symptoms in order to focus pharmacotherapy on the most burdensome of these. Optimal drug management could potentially improve the quality of care for people with dementia at the end of life. Consequentially, it is important to revise the therapeutic objectives of each comorbid disease and adapt treatments accordingly – withdrawing medications in a stepwise manner to assess

adverse reactions and impact on symptom profile. The withdrawal of acetylcholinesterase inhibitors is however a debatable area and more research is needed to support their discontinuation in late- to end-stage dementia.

Advance care planning and bereavement issues for people with advanced dementia and their families

It is of particular importance that people with dementia are supported, maintained and cared for until death in the environment of their choice and with the support of family members. Loss of decision-making capacity is a hallmark of dementia, and as in many cases the duration of the illness is prolonged, the supportive care demands placed on family or significant others may escalate over time.

To engage in advance care planning requires the person with dementia and their families to have some insight and understanding of the dementia illness trajectory. But evidence shows that this insight and understanding is generally lacking. Consequently, uncertainty and distress related to decision-making processes in preparation for the death of a person with dementia is often experienced by family members and significant others, and can have a negative impact on bereavement experiences.

Initiation of discussions about death and dying should take place at an early assessment stage, when the person with dementia can participate meaningfully in any discussion about death and dying with their families and caregivers. It is often assumed that 'surrogate' (family members or significant others) are fully cognisant of the treatment preferences of the person with dementia but this is not always the position. Shared decision-making with family and health professionals is essential, in order to provide care in a person's best interests, often for symptomatic relief rather than cure. Surrogate decision-makers may have taken out a Lasting Power of Attorney, or may need to approach the Court of Protection to take on the authority to act on the person's behalf in relation to health and financial affairs (see Chapter 12).

Challenges faced by families of people with late-stage dementia are unfamiliarity with death and lack of understanding of the natural course of late-stage dementia. An increased level of support may be needed. Historically, families of people with dementia have rarely received comprehensive bereavement services. The nature of

---

ABC of Dementia, First Edition. Edited by Bernard Coope and Felicity Richards.
© 2014 John Wiley & Sons, Ltd. Published 2014 by John Wiley & Sons, Ltd.

bereavement is complex and may be different at various stages as a dementia progresses.

Risk factors for mortality in dementia

A person with dementia may have up to five (or more) comorbid illnesses that could potentially be the cause of their death; however, there is little information on survival patterns and causes of death for people with dementia. Most studies have shown some evidence that there is lower survival for people with dementia in an institution rather than in the community. At best, research studies have identified risk factors that will contribute to death for specific dementia syndromes (Box 13.1).

Box 13.1 Progress and causes of death in the four main types of dementia

Alzheimer's disease (AD)	Impairment of person's basic bodily functions (swallowing, weight loss, loss of muscle strength, immobility)
	Significantly increased risk of developing pneumonia
	Pneumonia most commonly idaentified cause of death in AD
Vascular dementia	Progress of neurological changes is erratic
	Death usually due to cardiac or cerebral 'event'
Dementia with Lewy bodies (DLB)	Severe/advanced dementia and immobility (a few patients progress very rapidly through the disease)
	As with AD, pneumonia is typically the cause of death
Frontotemporal dementia (FTD)	Late-stage FTD symptoms include a gradual reduction in speech, culminating in mutism, failure or inability to make motor responses, akinesia (loss of muscle movement) and rigidity
	Death due to complications of immobility, most commonly pneumonia
	FTD progresses more rapidly than AD

Data from Alzheimers Association (2013) and Kohl (2011).

The Gold Standards Framework provides clinical prognostic indicators to identify people with dementia who are in need of supportive and palliative care (Box 13.2). These indicators are designed to be used when people may die within the next 6–12 months; however, prognostication in non-cancer patients is not generally precise. Factors usually associated with shorter survival in advanced dementia include severe cognitive impairment, parietal lobe dysfunction, dysphasia, psychotic symptoms, behavioural abnormalities, physical incapacity and poor nutrition.

Mortality and morbidity are significantly increased in the presence of other illnesses such as pneumonia (possibly as a result of compromised swallowing), sepsis as a result of other infections (e.g. pressure ulcers and urinary tract infections (UTIs)), cachexia, dehydration, cardiac disease and cerebral vascular disease. Mortality in the 6 months after the development of swallowing and feeding problems is significantly increased.

Box 13.2 Clinical prognostic indicators: patients with frailty and dementia

- Unable to walk without assistance and
- Urinary and faecal incontinence and
- No consistently meaningful verbal communication and
- Unable to dress without assistance
- Barthel score < 3

Plus any one of the following:
 Ten percent weight loss in previous 6 months without other causes, pyelonephritis or UTI, serum albumin < 25 g/L, high Waterlow score for pressure sore risk, recurrent fevers, reduced oral intake/weight loss, aspiration pneumonia.

Gold Standards Framework Centre (2011)

Symptoms experienced by people with dementia at the end of life

People dying with dementia have symptoms and health care needs comparable with those with cancer (Box 13.3) but experience these symptoms for much longer because of the often slow progression of their illness. Furthermore, people with dementia are at risk of over-treatment with burdensome and possibly non-beneficial interventions as well as under-treatment of symptoms (van der Steen, 2010), which, if addressed, would improve their end-of-life experiences.

Box 13.3 Most common symptoms experienced by people with dementia at end of life

Pain	Infections
Swallowing difficulties	Dehydration
Breathlessness	Cachexia
Acute confusion/delirium	Anxiety/fear/depression
	Constipation

Pain

Pain is under-reported and under-treated for people with dementia. As dementia progresses, there is a decline in cognitive function and the ability to verbally communicate. Loss of communication presents a major challenge in accurately assessing pain experienced by people with dementia. A useful and effective approach in pain assessment is to enlist the assistance of a caregiver or family member who is familiar with the usual behaviours and responses of the person with dementia and identify changes in behaviour that may indicate pain or discomfort.

In the absence of verbal self-report, increasing reliance is placed on non-verbal and behavioural cues that indicate the presence of pain. A combination of indicators to determine presence and levels of pain are shown in Box 13.4.

Box 13.4 Possible indicators of pain

Facial grimacing	Increased heart rate, blood pressure or sweating	Lethargy or increased sleep
Gestures that indicate distress		Disrupted or restless sleep
Guarding a particular body part or reluctance to move	Restlessness	Decreased appetite (and decreased nutritional intake)
	Crying or distress	
	Increased or decreased vocalisations	
Moaning with movement		Increased confusion
Limited range of motion or slow movement	Withdrawn social behaviour	Anger, aggression, irritability

Review of Tools for Assessment of Pain in Nonverbal Older Adults http://prc.coh.org/PAIN-NOA.htm

---

A large number of pain assessment tools have been developed for people with dementia. A sample of these are presented in Table 13.1; however, it remains a complex area of clinical practice. It is important to select a scale that matches the person's abilities including pre-morbid abilities, intelligence and educational level as these influence the individual's ability to respond to assessment.

Following assessment and identification of pain, it is imperative that pain is effectively managed. The World Health Organization (WHO) (1986) Analgesic Ladder (Figure 13.1) provides a framework for managing pain in palliative care that has sound applicability to managing pain in dementia care.

The principles within the framework are that the most appropriate analgesic is administered at a dose that relieves pain without causing

Table 13.1 A selection of pain assessment tools for people with cognitive impairment.

Tool	Full title
ABBEY	ABBEY Pain Scale
ADD	Assessment of Discomfort in Dementia
CNPI	Checklist on Nonverbal Pain Indicators
DBS	Discomfort Behavior Scale
Dis DAT	Disability Distress Assessment Tool
DS-DAT	Discomfort Scale-Dementia of the Alzheimer's Type
Doloplus 2	Doloplus 2
NOPPAIN	Nursing Assistant-Administered Instrument to Assess Pain in Demented Individuals
PAINAD	Pain Assessment in Advanced Dementia

Data from Review of Tools for Assessment of Pain in Nonverbal Older Adults http://prc.coh.org/PAIN-NOA.htm

unmanageable side effects (Table 13.2), combined with the administration of appropriate adjuvants (co-analgesics) (Table 13.3).

Adjuvant analgesics are drugs that do not function primarily as analgesics to relieve pain but can act to relieve pain in specific circumstances. For people with dementia, the 'usual' list of adjuvants needs to be extended to include therapeutic interventions that have been shown to be beneficial in dementia care practice (Therapeutic column – Table 13.3).

Swallowing difficulties

Oropharyngeal dysphagia, which leads to the person's inability to swallow food or fluids, becomes a major issue in late-stage dementia. This can be a very challenging condition for families and caregivers, regularly leaving them feeling helpless with the belief that providing food for the person is at least 'doing something'. Discussions regarding sustenance technology or artificial hydration and nutrition should take place at this stage and are often emotive, controversial and are influenced by complex ethical, religious, cultural and legal questions.

The General Medical Council (GMC) (2008) provides a framework for good practice for these processes in the 'Consent guidance: patients and doctors making decisions together' publication (www.gmc-uk.org). The most important consideration is to establish what is in the person's best interests, and whether there is

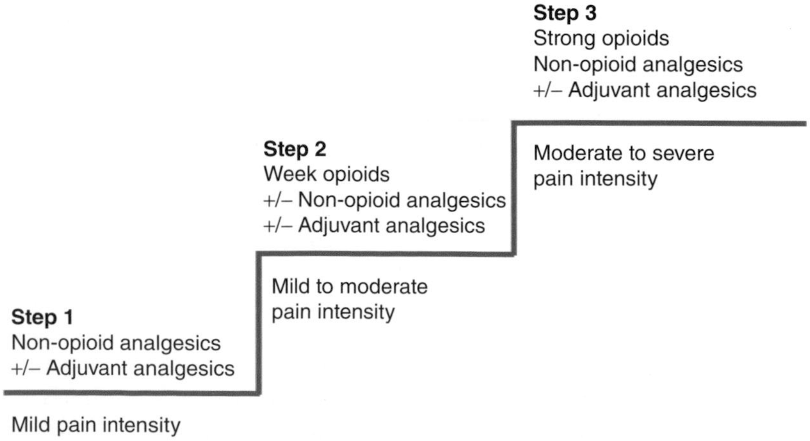

Step 3
Strong opioids
Non-opioid analgesics
+/– Adjuvant analgesics

Moderate to severe pain intensity

Step 2
Week opioids
+/– Non-opioid analgesics
+/– Adjuvant analgesics

Mild to moderate pain intensity

Step 1
Non-opioid analgesics
+/– Adjuvant analgesics

Mild pain intensity

Figure 13.1 The Analgesic Ladder. WHO (1986).
Reproduced by permission of World Health Organization

Table 13.2 Principles for the correct use of analgesics.

The oral form of medication should be favoured whenever possible
Analgesics should be given at regular intervals
The dosage of medication should be adjusted until the person is comfortable
Prescribe the dosage to be taken at definite intervals in accordance with the person's level of pain
Prescribe in accordance to pain intensity as evaluated by a scale of intensity of pain
Dosing of pain medication should be adapted to the person (the correct dosage is one that will allow adequate relief of pain)
Regularity of analgesic administration is crucial for the adequate treatment of pain
Analgesics should be prescribed with a constant concern for detail

Data from Vargas-Schaffer (2010).

Table 13.3 Adjuvant analgesics.

Therapeutic	Medications	Physical interventions
Music therapy	Non-steroidal anti-inflammatory drugs (NSAIDs)	Transcutaneous electrical nerve stimulation (TENS)
Relaxation therapy	Anticonvulsants	Acupuncture
Comforting and distraction	Muscle relaxants	Chiropractic
Therapeutic touch	Antidepressants	Physiotherapy and physical therapy
Gentle massage (hands)	Steroids	Local anaesthetics
Aromatherapy	Antispasmodics	Surgical and neurosurgical procedures
Minimising sensory overstimulation	Antibiotics	
	Compounds that act synergistically with opioids such as cannabinoids (e.g. nabilone)	

Data from Leung (2012), Vargas-Schaffer (2010), and Douglas et al. (2004).

an Advance Decisions to Refuse Treatment (ADRT) in place. There is no evidence that tube feeding or a percutaneous endoscopic gastrostomy (PEG) improves survival, functional status or comfort.

At a practical level, when the person becomes unable to swallow, is vomiting, has severe weakness or is unconscious, medications that are essential to maintain comfort may be administered via a subcutaneous syringe driver or via the rectal route. This is of particular importance if the person with dementia had required certain medications to control distressing symptoms, such as pain, before losing the ability to swallow or becoming unconscious. Medications that are not essential to the comfort of the patient at end

of life should be discontinued. However, death from pneumonia may cause great suffering and antibiotics (a recognised adjuvant analgesic on the WHO Analgesic Ladder; see Table 13.3) may be used to decrease discomfort even when death is imminent.

Dehydration and cachexia

Dehydration for people with dementia may arise when it becomes obvious that the person can no longer swallow. Some studies suggest that cachexia/dehydration is a more common cause of death than bronchopneumonia for people who survive to the final phase of dementia. Furthermore, evidence would suggest that withholding food and fluids in people with dementia with intake difficulties at the end of life does not cause undue discomfort.

Acute confusion/delirium superimposed on dementia

Delirium superimposed on dementia is common among older patients along their illness path but also near the end of life. Delirium can be triggered by a number of events such as infection, medications, dehydration, constipation, falls, a noisy environment and moving to a new or different environment. It is associated with a range of adverse outcomes such as accelerated cognitive and functional decline, longer hospital admissions and increased readmission, institutionalisation and death. The use of sedation in the event of delirium needs to be carefully considered, particularly the use of antipsychotics. Careful assessment will enable the identification of the cause of agitated behaviour related to delirium and therapeutic management of this must also be considered (see Table 13.3), Edwards (2003).

Infections

At the end of life, people are particularly vulnerable to infections. Prolonged physical immobility increases the risk of pressure sores, causes reduced coughing and deep breathing and increases susceptibility to pneumonia. Incontinence and catheterisation increase the risk of development of UTIs. It is not easy to identify the cause of infection in people with dementia as fevers can also be caused by conditions such as constipation or transient dehydration. The use of antibiotics to treat infections in severe dementia is controversial; however, on the basis of palliative care principles, a broad spectrum antibiotic is appropriate in many cases. Decisions to administer need to be judged on an individual's specific circumstances.

Conclusion

End-of-life care for people with dementia and their families is complex and multifaceted. A conservative or palliative approach to care is the preferred pathway. Maintaining comfort and dignity is a primary goal, keeping in mind that the terminal stages of dementia are difficult to predict. Such an approach needs to consider weighing the discomfort of the experience of being taken from familiar surroundings, against a hospital admission where that person may be subject to invasive medical interventions. Family members are most likely to remember events of the last days of life and these can significantly impact on their bereavement experiences. It is important that relevant discussion is initiated and clear explanations given in relation to care, so that decisions can be shared – preventing anxieties from lack of understanding of the dying process. It is considered good practice to reassure relatives that they have made the right decisions regarding any interventions or non-intervention related to care.

References

Edwards, N. Differentiating the 3D's: delirium, dementia and depression. MEDSURG Nursing 2003;**12**(6):347–357.

van der Steen, JT. Dying with dementia: What we know after more than a decade of research. J Alzheimer Dis 2010; **22**:37–55.

Alzheimers Association. *2012 Alzheimer's Disease Facts and Figures, Alzheimer's & Dementia*, **8**(2). 2013. http://www.alz.org/downloads/facts_figures_2012.pdf (accessed November 2013).

Kohl H, Special Committee on Aging. *Alzheimer's Disease and Dementia: A Comparison of International Approaches.* 2011. http://www.aging.senate.gov/reports/rpt2012.pdf (accessed November 2013).

Leung L. From ladder to platform: a new concept for pain management. *J Prim Health Care* 2012; **4**(3):254–258.

Vargas-Schaffer G. Is the WHO analgesic ladder still valid? *Can Fam Phys* 2010;**56**(6):514–517.

Douglas S, James, I, Ballard, C. Non-pharmacological interventions in dementia. *Adv Psych Treat* 2004;**10**:171–179.

World Health Organization (WHO). *Cancer Pain Relief*. 1986. https://extranet.who.int/iris/restricted/bitstream/10665/43944/1/9241561009_eng.pdf (accessed November 2013).

Herr K; Bursch H; Black B, et al. *State of the Art Review of Tools for Assessment of Pain in Nonverbal Older Adults* 2006. http://prc.coh.org/PAIN-NOA.htm (accessed November 2013).

Gold Standards Framework Centre. *GSF Prognostic Indicator Guidance.* 2011 http://www.goldstandardsframework.org.uk/cd-content/uploads/files/General%20Files/Prognostic%20Indicator%20Guidance%20October%202011.pdf (accessed November 2013).

Index